Memories linger on

yes. Suzy

ALL MY YESTERDAYS

ALL MY YESTERDAYS

by

SATYA CHATTERJEE

The Memoir Club

© Satya Chatterjee 2006

First published in 2006 by
The Memoir Club
Stanhope Old Hall
Stanhope
Weardale
County Durham

British Library Cataloguing in
Publication Data.
A catalogue record for this book
is available from the
British Library

ISBN: 1 84104 099 1

Typeset by TW Typesetting, Plymouth, Devon
Printed by CPI Bath

Dedication

To Ruth, Tom and Nicholas

Contents

List of Illustrations   ix

Foreword   xi

Acknowledgements   xiii

Chapter 1   Memories out of the dust   1

Chapter 2   Medical college   14

Chapter 3   In the army   24

Chapter 4   Days of decision   36

Chapter 5   The great adventure   47

Chapter 6   Newcastle and Manchester   56

Chapter 7   An American fellowship   67

Chapter 8   Baguley and Wythenshawe Hospitals   75

Chapter 9   Continental travel   84

Chapter 10 Gandhi Hall   93

Chapter 11 Return to India   102

Chapter 12 Recognition   108

Chapter 13 The Overseas Doctors' Association   118

Chapter 14 The medico-political world   126

Chapter 15 Towards retirement   134

Chapter 16 A debt of gratitude   143

Chapter 17 The last syllable   153

List of Illustrations

Granddaughter Ruth playing hide-and-seek in Woollaton
  Park 2

The author's mother 5

The author (right) with his brothers (back row), his father,
  sister and grandparents (middle row) and his nephews and
  nieces 10

Dr K. P. Bhargava in 1949 29

Dr Shanta Bhargava in 1949 30

The author (left) in America with Dr Lingapa and (front) Dr
  Ericson 72

Camille (left), Petula and Nigel in Heaton Moor, Stockport,
  Cheshire, in 1958 91

The author with Dr Shanta Bhargava 105

With Petula at St Andrews University 107

The author (left) with Dr Venogopal (right) and Dr Karim
  Admani 124

The author (right) in his garden with (left) Dr K. P.
  Bhargava and Dr Shanta Bhargava in 1981 131

The author in his room at Wythenshawe Hospital 136

The author with Ruth and Tom in 1992 141

The author with grandson Nicholas aged 8 at his Prep
  School on Prize-giving Day 144

Nigel and his wife Fran in their garden in Bermuda 144

(left to right) Dr Patrick Knowlson, Enid, Mrs Nora
  Knowlson, the author 146

The author and Enid in the garden of Dr Shanta Bhargava's
  home in New Delhi 147

The author lecturing at a medical symposium in 1995 . . . 150

In Bikaner with participants in the 1999 CME programme 151

The author with Enid, Petula, and Shanta Bhargava at the
    Taj Mahal in February 2005 155

The author's brother, Sona Chatterjee 155

Ruth at Liverpool University after her graduation in 2000 158

Tom's graduation from Sheffield University in 2001: (from
    left) Tom's father Paul, the author, Tom, Ruth, Enid .. 159

Nicholas and his grandparents after his graduation from
    Nottingham University in 2004 159

A family group: (from left) Enid, Camille, the author,
    Nicholas, Ruth, Tom, Petula, Paul 160

Foreword

This autobiography spans the latter two thirds of the twentieth century. As well as telling a fascinating personal story, it indirectly provides a social and cultural commentary on changes in the medico-political background in the UK of the times. The author, Dr Satya Chatterjee, a very well-known figure in respiratory medicine and research, after qualifying in India and after a broad medical development, was for many years a Consultant Chest Physician in the Manchester area. He is equally well-known for his tireless work for those who were then termed Overseas Doctors, of whom, at the time he was active, there were over 20,000 working in the National Health Service – a very significant body of professionals. With an enormous capacity for hard work, and so ably supported by his wife, Enid, his open-mindedness, fairness, and effortless grasp of complex situations brought him into great demand for public service in different capacities, and this was complemented by his medical distinction in elected membership of the General Medical Council and other bodies. His major contributions to the community in general, and to race relations in particular, were recognised in 1971 by the award of an OBE.

As a founder member and longserving officer of the Overseas Doctors' Association, he, and his wife and family, with their fellow officers and families, supported over sixty divisions of the ODA nationally, participating in their many local meetings and other events in which involvement of the families was a crucial aspect. Naturally, they have a very wide circle of friends, complementing their family of three, one of whom is medically qualified.

Satya Chatterjee is characteristically modest about his experiences and achievements in fields and times of unusual interest, with honest observations, insight, humour, and a fund of interesting anecdotes. This period saw the evolution of a large number of doctors originating overseas into settled UK citizens, with different issues of concern. They will be able to reflect on the contribution by the author, and his like-minded colleagues, in a formative period of great significance for this group of British doctors.

The background to his personal journey has thus been historically eventful. However, the author has never seemed concerned with destiny, always seeking in an emerging situation to do the best possible for the greatest overall good. In this way, events are guided along, rather than ends pre-shaped. With his youthful attitude, allied to the wisdom and judgement of age enriched by medical practice, one hopes that further experiences in his continuing journey may be recorded in due course.

Patrick Knowlson, M.D.

Acknowledgements

The title is not mine – borrowed from William Shakespeare as are bits of his poetry here and there in the book.

I am grateful to the Memoir Club and especially Eileen Finlayson for her encouragement and guidance and to Enid for her help, criticism and support and for typing.

I would like to thank Shiv Sherma for his tireless effort and patience in help with the preparation and manuscript.

I must also thank my old friend Patrick Knowlson for agreeing to write the Foreword, and for the friendship we have had over the years.

Of course my thanks go to my family – my children Camille, Petula and Nigel who have been an encouragement and inspiration in my many activities. The grandchildren Ruth, Tom and Nicholas who kept me up to date with the errors in the manuscript.

CHAPTER 1

Memories out of the dust

THE LITTLE BLONDE GIRL, her face a picture of milk-fed innocence, puts her young, gloved hand into mine for support and playfully kicks the dry, fallen leaves with her foot as a soccer player kicks a football, scattering scores of them in all directions. She is full of the joys of spring, although it's the beginning of autumn. The sky is blue and there is plenty of warmth in the air. The two of us are having an afternoon stroll in Nottingham's Woollaton Park. We both walk with unhurried steps, slowly, leisurely. She is my granddaughter, Ruth Periton – my daughter's daughter.

I have come from Wilmslow, Cheshire, to visit my daughter and her family in Nottingham. I have just had a big lunch, slightly later than my usual time, and am feeling quite relaxed. I am in a state of mind that's very sleep-inducing. But instead of having a shut-eye, I decide to take a walk. Ruth wants to accompany me so she quickly gets ready. She is well wrapped and has Clark's shoes on her young feet.

'Grandee, did you have a grandfather?' asks Ruth sweetly.

'Oh yes, I had a grandfather,' I tell her.

'And a grandmother?'

'And a grandmother.'

'What was she like, Grandee?'

'Like your grandmother,' I say after some thought. 'Well, like any grandmother, really . . . warm, affectionate, caring, with lots and lots of patience. You need a lot of patience, you know, when you've grandchildren. And I loved my grandma. We all loved her, my brothers and sisters.'

She seems quite pleased with my reply and her attention wanders either to something else that she has spotted in the park or by a thought that has found its way into her mind. She smiles and goes quiet. Unusual.

'Were you naughty sometimes?' Ruth looks up and asks me, with a hint of mischief in her eyes.

'When we were, my grandmother chastised us. You know, she told us off in no uncertain terms. Occasionally, very occasionally, she punished us. Not to hurt or harm us, but to make us better . . . to teach us what was wrong and what was right so that when we grew up we'd be a credit to our family, our country, and only do things that were right. You understand?'

She nods her young head in which, I can guess, a lot of things are milling around with each other. The mind-mill is in good working order and operating in top gear. From the expression on her face it's clear she is reassured that all children can be naughty at times.

A bunch of youngsters on roller-blades skate past us at some speed. One of them has a personal stereo. As he is not plugged in, it is pouring out music into the air loudly. It derails my train of memories. It all happens very suddenly. One minute they are there, the next minute they're gone. Ruth seems not to mind them at all. In fact, she looks quite pleased by the 'disturbance'. She is even softly humming a part of the song she has just heard.

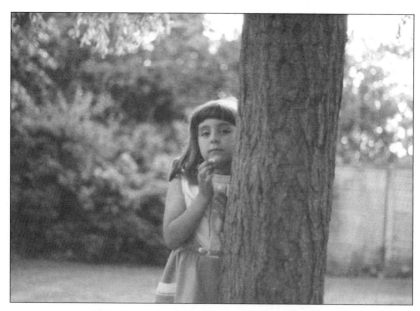

Granddaughter Ruth playing hide-and-seek in Woollaton Park

She has a good sense of rhythm and is nodding her head. Ah well, I sigh to myself, my loss is her gain.

'Are you warm enough, my little poppet?' I ask Ruth, as it is beginning to get a little nippy and also because she has not spoken for some time.

'Yes, Grandee,' she replies softly, without looking up, and continues to walk. 'I'm fine.' It seems she has nothing to ask me – for the time being at least. But I can almost hear that she is turning things over in her mind. She is bound to ask one thing or another soon, I'm sure of that.

A dog comes charging in our direction, panting and puffing and furiously wagging its tail. Ruth moves closer to me. She is an animal lover and is not frightened but it's the speed with which the dog approaches that alarms her a little. Within no time its owner arrives, telling the excited dog to calm down. I exchange a few words with him, mostly of a complimentary nature to his pet.

Ruth asks for permission to stroke the dog and he gives it immediately. She takes her hand out of the glove and warmly runs it over the dog's head three or four times, saying something to the animal. To show its affection, the dog stands on its hind legs for a moment and tries to smell her coat with its wet nose while offering a paw in friendship. The man says how pleasant the day is and I readily agree with him. He departs, the dog running ahead of him.

I hear the sound of an ice-cream van in the distance and think young Ruth will be interested in a choc bar or something. But she seems not bothered. Perhaps she has not heard the musical notes from the van. I am really surprised.

'Did you hear what I heard just now?' I ask her, probing while also playing a guessing game with her.

'What, Grandee?' she demands.

'The ice-cream van?'

'I did,' she nods.

'Do you want a lolly or a choc bar then?'

She thinks for a time.

'Let's do this. We'll go there and if it's still there we'll get one.'

'Will you have one as well?'

'Sure.'

She's pleased with the idea – something to look forward to. She skips and jumps a little.

Kicking the dead leaves in a park or wood is such clean, innocent fun and a favourite activity of children. It comes almost naturally to them, as though it were a part of their system, like eating, drinking and playing. We have had a long dry spell and there has been no rain for several days. The ground is biscuit-dry. She plays a little hopscotch and kicks the leaves again. A little dust rises into the air as she does that.

Ruth and I slowly trudge on our way. The ice-cream van is there but the salesman is gathering his things and preparing to leave. I think another couple of minutes and we would've missed him. He has no lollies or cones left. The business on that autumn day must have been good. Ruth has to settle for a choc bar and I take a tub, vanilla-flavoured. As we leave the park, she gives the fallen leaves one final kick.

I glance down casually and see a lot of dust rising. The foot that raises the dust this time is mine and it has Bata's canvas shoes on. Between the two is a chasm, deep with years – as many as it takes one from *having* a grandfather to *being* a grandfather.

It's so mixed with memories, this kicking of leaves. Suddenly I recall how, a long time ago, I used to kick leaves, stones, bottle-tops, virtually anything, really, that lay on the road on my way to the mangroves to play cricket with my friends. The place was Patna, in India's Bihar state.

I was born into a middle-class family in Calcutta, recently renamed as Kolkatta, and was one of five children – three brothers and two sisters. Our ancestral home was not very far away. It was in a village called Rahuta, about twenty miles south of the city. My grandfather worked in Calcutta Secretariat. It was also the place where my father was employed. My parents moved to Patna, in the neighbouring state of Bihar, when a new secretariat opened there. We had a house in Gardanibagh, a dormitory town, well planned, well ordered, with schools, gardens, roads and other civil amenities. Although we were not rich, we were reasonably well off, able to get all the things we needed for a comfortable living.

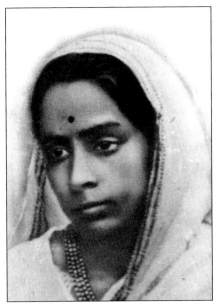

The author's mother

My parents looked after us well and we were happy in our new house. I was in primary school when my mother took ill. My grandparents came from Calcutta to look after her. But she did not get better. One day there was a lot of commotion in the house and a body covered in a shroud was carried out. All those present were crying and consoling each other amid tears that streamed down their faces. Everyone was sad. I was, too, without realizing the finality of my loss. After my mother was cremated, my grandparents stayed behind to look after us. In the absence of a mother, my grandmother took the role of bringing us up and had a great influence on me. She was kind and generous, always coming round to see us at night to make sure we were nicely tucked in bed. She brought a glass of milk that she put by our bedside and told us not to fall asleep without drinking it and returned a few minutes later to see that we had finished it.

As the years passed, my father got promoted at work and this resulted in our moving to a bigger place, which was to be our home for the next twelve or thirteen years. The house had three bedrooms and a garden. It was close to a secondary school, which I was later to attend myself. The school was the biggest I had seen so far in my young life. It had a huge playground, a gymnasium and drill room. Our headmaster, Dr Ashutosh Ghattak, was a very strict person. Discipline in those days, I think, was considered to be very important and a vital part of a child's education and upbringing. In those days I thought the headmaster was too strict. He belonged to the spare-the-rod-and-spoil-the-child school of thought. Hardly surprising, therefore, that he was always armed with a cane when he went on his daily round of the school or was just spotted in the corridors on his way from one place to another. If any pupil was found loitering or in any way out of step with the rules of behaviour, he was ready to dispense his brand of justice. I had good reason to fear him because I wasn't particularly good at studies. I had difficulty with some subjects and English spelling. But I was hardworking. What I lacked by way of talent, I made up with industry. I just wanted to get on with my education. I suspect that I may have had a mild form of dyslexia, a condition which at that time was not recognised.

I do not remember the wedding of my elder sister as I must have been very young at the time, or probably was not keen on matters that mainly concerned the elders of the family. Maybe they had decided I was not grown up enough to be assigned any responsible task connected with the wedding. But the marriage of my second sister is fresh in my mind to this day, although it took place more than half a century ago. She was married in Calcutta. My father booked two second-class train carriages from Patna. He rented a house in the Sibpur district of the city where the marriage ceremony took place. I remember we youngsters had a thunderously good time. Weddings in India are big, and some-times lavish, affairs. All the relatives came from faraway places.

On the day of the wedding, four cars, full of guests including the bridegroom, arrived. We stood outside the house in our new clothes to welcome them, teeth gleaming, shoes shining. My impression was that they were nice people, pleasant, smartly attired, and they seemed undemanding. We put them up in a room fully carpeted and tastefully decorated. The servants brought sweets, savouries, fruit, and drinks made with yoghurt. The groom went with my father and the ladies to a marquee where the wedding ceremony was to take place. He sat with all his relatives. We youngsters were curious, like newly hatched chicks, to see what was happening. The ceremony proceeded at a slow pace, as Indian weddings often do. My sister looked very pretty in her wedding dress and make-up.

For some unknown reason, these ceremonies in India, particularly Bengal, begin at night – the later the better. I guess it's because the days are extremely hot. And they go on well into the early hours. The priest started reciting the mantras, and administered marriage vows with great solemnity to the couple, who went round the sacred flame to conclude the ceremony. The newly-weds were served food at a place specially reserved for them. It had a little bit of privacy. There was plenty of music, singing and dancing. This bit of the celebration was not organised beforehand. There were no dress rehearsals, no practice rounds, no pre-assigned roles. It was all very impromptu, spur-of-the moment stuff. Things just happened. But it went off quite well. All my visiting cousins took part in the goings-on. It was a very jolly occasion.

One character I cannot forget at my sister's wedding was a friend of my father. On the wedding day, he came very early to our house and had a brief conference with my father and others involved with the organisation of the event. Having ensured everything was well in hand, he headed straight to the kitchen where, for the rest of the day, he was up to his elbows in work, cleaning the fish, chopping it, frying it and cooking it, then turning his attention to other things. He also lent a hand where a hand was needed and generally kept a watchful eye on those who were busy with other preparations. Then, as the sun went down, he emerged from the kitchen, had a quick drench bath, a quick change of clothes and was ready to perform the duties of the priest. He did both jobs with great aplomb. He was also a very strict person – mostly with himself – because later I heard him say that he did all this without putting as much as a single morsel of food in his mouth. There was no religious sanction behind it. No rules of any other kind. He just did not want to eat until his ceremonial duties were over. He wanted to make certain that all the guests were properly looked after and fed on time and fed well. It was, according to him, very important in a Hindu family wedding.

Two days later, my sister went to her new home to start her married life and we returned to Patna to resume ours. Soon I was to experience the first natural disaster of my life. A terrible earthquake shook Patna in 1934. We had just got home from school one afternoon when suddenly everything shook and started to sway. The water tower in front of our house swung from side to side and thousands of gallons of water came crashing down. Telegraph poles toppled over, buildings were reduced to rubble and many people were buried alive under the debris. For us youngsters it was very frightening. We did not go inside the house as it had suffered structural damage. My father hurried home from work as soon as he could to see that no harm had come to us. Once he had make sure we were all right, he decided to build a little straw hut in the garden so that we wouldn't have to sleep inside the house that night, because everyone feared there would be more tremors. The earthquake was the only topic of conversation in the days that followed and all kinds of stories about the havoc it had caused kept cropping up in conversation for quite a while.

India is a land of thousands of gods and myriads of semi-gods. Then there are deities, devis, devtas and holy men. Virtually all of them have a following. Almost everything is worshipped – from a phallus to a number of trees and animals. Hindus believe that everything has a place in nature's grand scheme and it should be allowed to perform the duty for which it was created. As such, one is never far away from festivities, celebrations and ceremonies. The start of every season is ushered with offerings of one thing or another. There are celebrations to mark the various phases of the moon. Different sets of prayers are chanted at sunrise and at sunset. At eclipse of the sun and noon alms are given to the poor. Some of the ceremonies are of a personal nature, like a child's first haircut, which usually comes within the first year of the birth in most parts of the country. Then there is the cutting of the teeth, uttering of the first word. They all have their place in the great calendar of life.

I have no recollection of the early ones. But I certainly remember very well my sacred thread ceremony. It marks a youngster's entry into adulthood and usually comes in the early teenage years. To my brother and me it came when we were around fourteen or fifteen years of age. A joint function was organised for both of us. We made our way to the local river and had a bath. Upon our return, while a pundit recited prayers and chanted mantras for one and all to hear, we were ushered into a room where there wasn't much light. Each of us was given a begging bowl in which all those visiting put gifts of money and presents. This went on for seven days. We weren't allowed to talk to anybody and were forbidden to see the sun. The only food we were allowed was cooked at home by a close relative. In our case it was our grandmother. On the seventh day we once again went back to the river where our heads were shaved. We had a bath and were given a sacred thread to be worn next to our skin. From that time onwards for the next twelve months, we were to observe total silence while eating and all our meals were to be vegetarian. We also had to pray every morning and night. Some parts of this discipline, I must confess, I did not find hard to observe but others I wasn't so sure of. Once or twice, quite inadvertently, I spoke out during my meal, only to see my plate disappear out of sight.

My sister came from Calcutta for the ceremony and stayed on because she was expecting a child – her fifth. One day she suddenly fell ill and was rushed to hospital. She never returned. The baby was saved and my grandparents were left to tend to her five children. Poor souls, they had brought five children up when my mother died and now the lightning had struck again. I bow my head to them in gratitude whenever I think of the sacrifices they made, first for me and my brothers and sisters and then for our nephews and nieces. May God rest their souls in peace!

The year 1936 was a difficult one for us. I managed to scrape through the final of my school exams. I had no high hopes to begin with, but even my modest expectations were not met. My one big hope: there will always be another time to galvanise myself and do much better. I was thinking of this 'another time' because I had already been granted admission to the local science college to study for my intermediate certificate.

Intermediate, as the word applies, is a sort of halfway house between school and the university. After intermediate you decide whether you want to study science or take up arts. If you choose

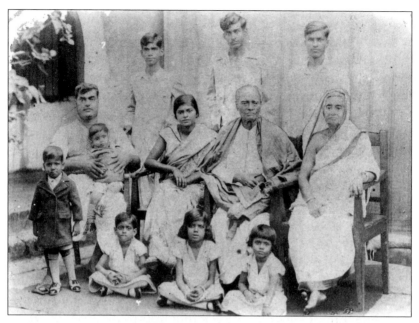

The author (right) with his brothers (back row), his father, sister and grandparents (middle row) and his nephews and nieces

the first, you get admitted to the science faculty and study for your Bachelor of Science degree, and if you opt for the latter you go to the arts side and prepare for the Bachelor of Arts degree. For a long time I was undecided what to choose. All I knew was, art or science, I wanted my studies to continue.

A friend of my father, who was a highly respected person in academic circles, suggested that if I took the science route and 'burnt the midnight oil by the gallon' I stood a good chance of being accepted in Patna Medical College, which, at the time, was one of the top medical colleges in India – easily among the top ten. As a gesture of encouragement my father bought me a spanking new bicycle so that I could ride to college on it. Owning a self-pushing, two-wheeled effort in those days was like having a power-packed, super-duper Ferrari today. I was thrilled to bits at having my own means of transport. Ah, the joys of pedal power! I really took good care of my bike, dusting it, washing it, wiping it to maintain its new look. To ring its bell suddenly while inches behind some poor, unsuspecting pedestrian, sending him or her into a state of temporary panic, was undiluted bliss – if kept within limits. I'm sure many an imprecation was directed silently at me in my carefree, youthful, cycling days.

The years at the science college were happy though uneventful. We had a lecturer who was keen to make us expert in English, while another believed that chemistry was a subject impossible to beat and wanted us to excel in it. Between the two they made sure that my English improved and my fondness for chemistry grew. Once again I passed, but once again the margin wasn't something to write home about in a hurry. Everyone thought that the marks I had obtained weren't high enough to earn me a place in Patna Medical College, which had only forty places. Out of these, two were reserved for girls and two for Muslims. There were further reservations for those belonging to scheduled castes and scheduled tribes. This left only a handful of places for the rest of the population, thereby making the competition all the more stiff. As uncertainty grew, dreams of rounds in hospital wards in a white coat with a stethoscope strung round my neck began to fade into the distance.

But I didn't completely give up. My hopes now rested on certain other factors, such as interviews and divine intervention. I even prayed to my guardian angel to blow the wind in my direction on the day of the selection. He seems to have heard me and answered my prayer when one morning I received a letter from the college asking me to attend an interview in the college library at 10.30 a.m. on a certain date. On the day of the interview I got up early in the morning. I scrubbed myself clean and put on clothes with razor-sharp ironing. The previous evening I had cleaned my bicycle — as if I would be allowed to take it into the interview room — and presented myself to the clerk of the college at least twenty minutes before time.

He was a rough sort of fellow, sharp and blunt of tongue. He raised a finger and pointed me to a stool, saying quite authoritatively, 'Take a seat over there.' Three other candidates had already been shown their places, no doubt in a similar fashion by him. All of us were nervous as hell and, from time to time, eyed each other sheepishly. The occasion was overwhelming and we didn't know what to do. Suddenly a peon appeared out of nowhere and announced my name loudly, as they do in a court of law when they summon a witness. Nervously, I dragged myself into the library. It was a daunting place, a semi-dark room, which in my nervous state looked completely dark to me. There was a large table at which, on tall chairs, sat four distinguished men in European clothes. They formed the selection committee. All seemed comfortable with themselves. One or two were smiling pleasantly at each other. One or two looked serious, even solemn. I heard a voice telling me to take a seat. I obeyed without a moment's hesitation. 'How old are you?' boomed a different voice.

'Seventeen, sir,' I stammered.

'Don't you think you're too young to be a medical student?' I offered no reply. Frankly, I didn't know what explanation to offer in defence of my age.

'You haven't done well, have you?' The same voice again but with little less boom. The man was looking at a piece of paper in front of him, apparently my science result, I figured.

'I know, sir,' I offered, admitting my not-so-good showing in the exam results.

'Your physics marks are low. You've barely scraped through,' my tormentor pressed on.

'The physics exam was very tough, sir,' I said weakly in my defence.

'No . . . no . . . that . . . that . . .'

How he completed the sentence I do not know. What I do know is that I made a quick assessment of my chances and they looked as dark as the room I was in.

The next person to address me was Professor Mohammed Husnan. He was the chairman of the selection committee and professor of Ear, Nose and Throat. He had heaps of personality and an imposing presence. The professor smiled before he spoke, 'Chatterjee, why do you want to be a doctor?' A thoughtful pause on my part. Then − what I thought was an inspired idea − I said in a voice full of conviction, 'To serve the suffering humanity, sir.' He drew back. Brave words from a young fella. I got the feeling he felt I meant it. I did. I still do.

I was not asked any questions by the next member of the committee, Col. Hugh Mahoney, a tall, burly, red-faced Englishman who was the superintendent of the college. He just smiled at me. What a relief! I relaxed. I was pleased I did not have to answer any questions from him. The voice of the clerk from one of the corners of the room told me that I could go and wait outside. I knew the place very well – one of the four stools. Of the four candidates that day one or two were told to go. I was one of those asked to remain available. It was difficult to read into it.

After a few agonising minutes the clerk emerged from the library and, with a smile the size of an unzipped banana, read the names of those who had been successful and I was among them. I immediately forgave him for his earlier crusty behaviour, thanked the harbinger of such good news three or four times with courteous little bows and left. I was so happy I did not know what to do with myself . . . skip, jump, run, do the cartwheel, shake hands with total strangers, slide down the college's balustrade, if it had one. In the end I hopped on my bicycle and rushed home to tell the good news that I had been accepted to study medicine at Patna Medical College, one of the top institutions in the country . . . certainly among the top ten.

My father was at work and my grandfather was having his afternoon siesta. I looked for my grandma and after some hurrying and scurrying found her in the kitchen. 'I've been accepted for entry into the college,' I said to her joyously.

'What does that mean?' she demanded, looking askance.

'I'm going to study medicine,' I screamed. 'I'm going to be a doctor.'

She gave me a look of bewilderment and said, 'You don't know what you're in for, my dear child.' She was right. I didn't. The next few years would tell me that.

CHAPTER 2

Medical college

THERE IS ONLY ONE WAY to describe Patna in July: an inferno. All the furnaces at the sun's disposal, big and small, are churning out heat at full throttle and they are, it certainly feels that way, trained on the city. From dawn to dusk, dry, dragon-breath winds prowl the streets unchallenged, keen to strike at anything and anybody that comes in their way. People try all kinds of folk recipes to ward off their effects and, should they by some chance fall victims to their merciless lash, to limit the damage.

At mid-day, the heat is so strong it softens the tar on the road.

When I learned that our education at Patna Medical College was to begin in July, I could not help feeling that the heat was truly on – both literally and metaphorically – but I was bubbling with enthusiasm and buoyed up by the feeling that would one day – all things proceeding to plan – put that coveted white coat on my back, a stethoscope round my neck and the all-important degree certificate on a wall in the lounge in an expensive frame. It had a music all its own, that four-letter degree, MBBS. In moments of day-dreaming, I used to close my eyes and see those letters, exquisitely engraved on a brass plate in capitals, announcing to the world at large that a doctor lives or works here. I would roll those letters round my tongue and savour them in my mouth. Dr S. S. Chatterjee, MBBS. I felt like rejoicing. The joy was unconfined!

One fine morning, the fateful day to begin my medical education arrived. Decked in spotless white clothes but nerves a-jangle, I arrived at the college on my bicycle to be met by thirty-seven others similarly attired, carrying the same dream in their heart. Some of them were as nervous as I was, others perhaps a bit less, still others perhaps a bit more. Also at work were a whole range of other emotions, like anticipation, curiosity, fear and heaven knows what else. Somewhere at the back of most minds was also the itching anxiety to find out about the two girls who would be our colleagues on the course. One, we soon found out, was an Anglo-Indian called Marie Quadros. The other was a Hindu by religion, and bore the name Sunder Devi. Naturally, we were eager to say hello to them, introduce ourselves to them and get to know them. But, being bashful, we just didn't have the courage to make the first move. I certainly kept postponing these formalities to a later date, when I was more settled in the course. After all, we were going to be together for years so where was the hurry! The important thing was that we had entered the college and taken our vows to heal a few, cure some and be compassionate to all. We were told – as if we didn't know it – that to accomplish this we needed the heart of a lion, the hands of a woman and the patience of Jove.

At that early stage, to our irritation, some members of the staff did not take us freshers with any seriousness, especially those with whom we had little contact. Each morning, we arrived at the college like knights in shining armour. There was a swagger in the way we walked, a cock-eyed over-confidence in the way we talked. Perhaps this is what did not go down well with them. They had, no doubt, seen it all many times before. We arrived punctually in the morning, attended the lectures, played football and returned home in the evening, nearly always whacked. We had found a new focus in life. We knew where we were going and were keen to get there.

Another item on our list of priorities was to meet other students, get to know them and sow the seeds of friendship with them. Medical colleges have always had a strong tradition of fraternity, brotherhood, group loyalty and so forth. I was no laggard in making friends or in influencing people. In the first few days I was one-fourth of a foursome, the other three being Sunil Bhattacharya, Sunil Chatterjee and Shibu Ghoshal. Whether it was lectures, science or mischief, we were always together, hunting in a pack. One area of common interest was to sit immediately behind the girls, who had their well-oiled, jet-black, streaming hair woven tightly into a plait or plaits, thick as a boxer's fists, which they left dangling behind them, the ends often resting blissfully on the desk immediately behind. The competition for those places was very intense indeed.

But whether seated behind the female students or elsewhere, we took a keen interest in the lectures. One lecturer, Dr Sanatan Pujari, who taught us anatomy, was just brilliant. A very experienced man, with bags of energy and warmth, he was thoroughly dedicated to his subject and he made sure what he offered enthusiastically was received with matching enthusiasm. I was awe-struck by his ability to dish out details of anatomy so facilely while he drew excellent pictures of parts of the human body on the blackboard with his left hand. To this day, his lectures on developmental anatomy and his blackboard drawings are deeply engraved on my mind. Another lecturer I greatly admired was Dr David Lacey. An Anglo-Indian, he taught us botany and biology. Besides these we also studied other subjects, including zoology, physiology and pharmacology in the first three years of our course. As friendships and fellowships were formed and cemented, there were plenty of extra-curricular activities to occupy our attention. One for which I had a particular liking was going down to the college's riverboat and rowing it early in the evening and occasionally in the afternoon, if the heat was not too strong. Nearly always, I returned home dog-tired but keen to attend the college the next day.

Exit MBBS part one after a university examination. I had crossed this hurdle without much fuss or worry. Our commitment to medicine was now taking roots and getting stronger with each passing day. Work was getting more demanding, life tougher as we had to sit for an examination at the end of each year. You just could not take your eyes off the syllabus ball. There were good days and bad days but all days were busy. The dissecting room was interesting, with long, frightening tables on which lay human parts in various stages of dissection. Students had to work in a team of two for each section of anatomy and my partner was Mansoor Alam. We soon became good friends and remained so for the next three years. We studied hard, drew our pictures diligently and, with a little help from my friend Sunil Bhattachar-jee, a cheery, enthusiastic fellow full of dash and energy, prepared a booklet. It was distributed to all the students of anatomy and was still in use long years after we graduated and bid farewell to the college.

Dr S. K. Ghosh was our senior lecturer in anatomy. He had returned to India after spending some time in England. A pleasant man, slightly on the plump side, he walked to the college every morning. Dr Ghosh was another of our teachers who made a deep impression on me. In my experience, students do well in a subject if they like the person who teaches it. So it was no surprise that, when the final result was declared, I had passed in anatomy with honours. As soon as the MBBS part two was over, we became clinical students. It was now time to start doctoring. We were lectured in medicine, surgery, obstetrics and gynaecology. These lectures were usually given in the morning and we did practical work in the afternoon. It was an exciting phase in our education, partly because it brought us into contact with patients and partly because it provided us with an opportunity to smile at the nurses and hope that they would reciprocate in similar fashion. Some of us were also able to flaunt our new status, showing off to relatives, non-medic friends and acquaintances that we were well and truly on our way to becoming fully-fledged, certified doctors.

In snow-white shirt and trousers, eyes twinkling, teeth gleaming and gelled hair, we lounged around the nurses' duty rooms, looking for a cup of tea – sugared with a smile, of course. I'm sure some of us cut a fine figure, because occasionally we did find a well-manicured female hand extending a cup of tea in our direction. However, we did not venture for dates at that stage, but hope was springing eternal. We were seeking friendships with nurses, medical colleagues and other members of the opposite sex working in the hospital. Some were even ready for a serious relationship.

One day, news broke that Mansoor Alam's parents were arranging his wedding. Nothing unusual about that, I suppose, except that if you're studying medicine you get it out of the way before taking a plunge into marital life. A newly-married wife, with all her hopes and dreams of romance, and a mind-numbing, time-consuming education, it seemed to most of us, did not make good bed-fellows. But what soon left everybody gasping for breath was the fact that the would-be bride was the daughter of another medical student, Murtaza Ahmed, who appeared slightly older than other students. On the due day, the marriage took place with great pomp and ceremony and we all attended.

At the beginning of the third year, I was given a room to myself in the hostel. The reason for this privilege was that I had been chosen as a prefect. Besides me there were five others picked for that special treatment. For the first few days it was a lonely existence, being on my own in the room with no one to talk to and discuss life and our education. So I asked one of the other foursome, Shibu Ghoshal, if he would like to share the accommodation with me. He leapt at the idea and was my room-mate for the next three years. Our friendship, though, went well beyond our college days.

Senior students exerted a lot of influence over us. They were a kind of role model for us. We admired them and looked up to them. After all, they were our peers. I don't think it was peer pressure in those days, more like peer influence. We needed it, too, especially when it came to creating some excitement in our lives, straying into mischief. One night, around 10.30 p.m. there was a knock on the door and there stood two of the seniors. They asked us to come out. We quietly obeyed. Within no time there were ten of us and we were going to row the college boat in moonlight. The plan was to make a lot of noise while rowing past the girls' hostel ... you know, shout and sing in a rowdy serenade, to attract their attention, to show them what a brave, clean and fun-loving lot we were.

The night was lovely. The moon was shining like a newly polished silver trophy. The plan was executed with military precision and it went off without a hitch. There was a lot of singing and dancing, laughing and cheering, whistling and clapping in the direction of the little rectangles of light in which stood the female of the species of the college. As we were returning to the mooring at midnight after the stunt, one of the senior students, Pashupati Laha, dared us to take off our clothes and streak from the riverbank to our hostel rooms, knowing full well that we'd have to pass through the main medical wards and almost certainly meet the changing of the shift for the nurses.

Just our luck. The first person we ran into was the night sister in her crisply starched uniform and white cap with all manner of clips and ribbons. The expression of horror that the sight of ten stark-naked young men, panting and puffing, brought to her face would have won any quick-clicking photographer top prize in a national competition. She screamed at the top of her voice, 'What the hell is going on here, boys?' Or words to that effect.

We spent the rest of the night giving ourselves a nervous breakdown. How would the authorities react when they came to know of us men behaving so badly? What would be our punishment? Thrown out of the college, perhaps? How were we going to explain it our parents? The damnations of hell were staring us starkly in the face. All sorts of frightening images flashed through our minds. But as it happened the night sister turned out to be a real sport. I think, after she had recovered from the brief encounter of the unclad kind with us, she saw the funny side of it and probably dismissed it all from her mind by saying to herself, 'Ah, well, boys will be boys.' Boys indeed! To our great surprise – and delight – we found in the next two or three days that no disciplinary action of any kind was forthcoming and we unanimously declared the night sister the Star of India.

Now imagine this scene. Two decades have passed. I am a lot older and a lot wiser. I am in the city of Gwalior, where I have a speaking engagement at a conference. Pashupati Laha, the chief architect of the nocturnal prank, is also there. He has really gone up in the world. He's a professor now. Professor Laha invites me to his house for a spot of fish-curry dinner and a trip down memory lane. I arrive at his house and press the front door bell. The door opens and I nearly have a cardiac arrest . . . for there, standing right in front of me, resplendent in a red sari and a matching dot on the forehead, is the night sister . . . now Mrs Laha. Simultaneously, we both burst into a Homeric laughter. The next day she invited me along with some of the other speakers for dinner, on the condition that dress would be informal – but essential. Three cheers to Mrs Laha.

While our medical education was proceeding at a steady pace, problems and tragedies were once again stalking my family. My father was diagnosed as having diabetes. This caused enormous worries to my grandparents because his eating habits were, to say the least, a bit wayward. Despite warnings, he was often seen gobbling sweetmeats in the office canteen at lunchtime. One evening I returned home to find the place eerily quiet. I soon discovered that our grandfather wasn't well. He was lying on the floor in one of the rooms because he found the bedding hot. The family doctor was sent for and arrived in no time. He carried out a quick examination and pronounced that there was nothing seriously wrong with the patient. The doctor scribbled out a prescription, gave a few words of advice on dos and don'ts and left.

A few hours after his departure, my grandfather's condition worsened. He just lay there without any movement. Around midnight he peacefully passed away. We sat at his feet quietly, our heads bowed in respect and gratitude for what he had done for us. He was a friend, he was a mentor, he was a guru and he was strict. But he was our granddad and we had lost him. We took his body to the cremation *ghat* and watched with tears in our eyes as it went up in flames. It was a sad and mournful house that we came back to. I lay down tired, exhausted and overcome by emotion. Next day, without being called, the family doctor arrived to have a look at his patient. He was shocked to hear the news. I could see it in his face. He froze up with the shock for a while. When he had regained his composure, he told us not to mourn our grandfather's death but to celebrate his life . . . think of how he had enriched our lives with his generosity, his good nature and his affection. Although we followed the doctor's advice, there was no escaping the fact that our grandfather's death had created an enormous void in our lives. Our grandmother was now the only beacon of light in our lives. Our father remained unapproachable, distant and aloof.

As time rolled on, studies continued apace and life was divided between college and home. Around 1942, my father fell ill with a serious inflammation at the back of his neck. Captain Pal, a well-known surgeon, came to see him and told us that he would have to be admitted to hospital for an operation. Although at that stage my medical knowledge was only limited, I pretended to know a hell of a lot more and took on a new role. With confidence, I told my brothers and relatives that it was the right thing to do and that surgery was the best course of action for our father. So we got him a separate room in the hospital and he underwent an operation there.

While all this was going on our grandmother kept complaining of not being well and she took to bed. Just three days later she peacefully passed away. What she was suffering from I do not know to this day, but I strongly suspect it was a broken heart. She was not the same person after her husband's death. My father was still in hospital at the time of her death. The final flame in our lives was put out.

With both our grandparents gone, I felt that we had no one left in the world. The sacrifices that my grandmother made for the family were enormous and were the hallmark of her life. First she had brought us up after my mother's death and then my sister left five of her children for her to care for. But, without a murmur of complaint on her lips or the furrow of a frown on her forehead, she looked after all of us with warmth and affection. As a naive child I used to think that people who had a lot of love to give never died. But they do. She did.

After this tragedy my father became a changed man. He was unhinged emotionally. Every morning he went to work. Every evening he came back home. But his interest in life, including the children, was minimal. I don't think life had dealt him a good hand. He lost his wife when he was young. Then he saw his daughter die, lost his parents, suffered ill health. Still in his forties, now his sons were ready to fly the coop. So many agonies. Such anguish. As I look back, sometimes I can empathise with him. There is often this gnawing feeling that we, father and sons, never really worked as a team. He had his responsibilities to the large family that we had become and the commitments of his job at the secretariat and we had our studies and our careers to think about and work towards. Somewhere between these two differing demands, no bonding took place and the closeness was lost.

Contrary to our mounting fears, the final exams were easy. A few weeks before they were due, senior students had a series of meetings with the lecturers. The idea was to winkle out any questions that they might have in their mind that they would use in the exam. I was chosen to do that for medicine because I knew the professor for that subject, T. N. Bannerjee, well. Particularly anxious to find out theoretical questions of mental health disease that none of us was keen to learn, I went to see him and asked, pretending as if it was just by the way, 'Sir, so far I haven't devoted much time to mental health diseases and was wondering if I should do so now?' His reply was that the subject was important and there were usually three questions on it in the exam. He wasn't giving anything away.

'Any particular part that could be considered of special interest?' I ventured, probing deeper. 'Acute depression is interesting, don't you think so?'

Pneumonia and diarrhoea were other topics that I had managed to worm out of the professor. Next morning, thanks to my highly skilful work, acute depression, pneumonia and diarrhoea were the talk of the student fraternity which was busy swotting for the exams.

Three weeks later we went to the senate hall to take them. We were given the question papers. Sure enough there was 'depression'. Turn the next page and the word 'pneumonia' appeared to my great delight, and what a treat it was to deal with the treatment of diarrhoea in summer. I was happy. I had served my fellow students and friends. In that examination hall, my stock must have shot up enormously in the eyes of my classmates. The only problem, however, was that everyone must have offered the same answer.

In the viva exam I was asked to judge an instrument. In a confident voice, I offered a long and detailed explanation. The trouble was I was prattling on about the wrong object. 'You've read the seven chapters of the holy book *Ramayana* and you say Sita was Rama's aunt?' Yes, I had badly boobed there. It must have cost me my honours in medicine. But happy ending or not-so-happy ending, I was pleased the exams were a memory.

We huddled together in front of the notice board on the day the results were declared. The list of the students who had been successful was posted there. Had I passed? That's all I wanted to know. What a huge relief it was to see my name. Yes, I had passed, and with honours in anatomy. I jumped up and looked around and wondered what it meant. Was I a doctor? Indeed I was. Another look round and I saw that others, too, had a similar expression on their faces.

With a spring in my step the like of which I had never experienced before, I made a mad dash for home. My father seemed unexcited by my achievement. 'Yes, I know,' he said in a businesslike manner. 'Had a phone call from the college.'

But this was not the sort of response I wanted from him. I wanted him to take my hand and shake it enthusiastically. I wanted him to congratulate me. I was hungry for a hefty 'well done' pat on the back. After all, it was no mean achievement to be the first doctor in the family. I wanted that fact to be recognised by everyone present.

As my brother was married now, his wife came into the room carrying a bowlful of *rasgoolas*, a sweet that drips with syrup and is a firm favourite of every Bengali. With a smile, she forced one into my mouth and quickly followed it with another.

So just two *rasgoolas* were my reward for six years of hard work. I felt I deserved better.

CHAPTER 3

In the army

HELLO LIFE, take me to your great adventure playground, I'm a doctor now.

This was the state of my euphoric mind in the first few days of qualifying and who could blame me! I was enthusiastic about things as they were and full of hopes about things to come. With a medical degree under my belt, I thought I was God's favoured co-pilot and when He went on holiday I would take over the controls. I'm sure even today graduates get that feeling when they pass their degree exam.

Life, though, had different, more realistic, designs for me. There was, to begin with, the small matter of doing my time in the Indian Army. During the final year of our medical education, the Inspector General of Civil Hospitals, Colonel John Speakman, had sent a circular asking the final year students to consider volunteering for the army and I had signed a contract to that effect. On offer from the army was a generous training allowance. The other carrot was an implied suggestion that a stint in khaki would carry weight for those who had successfully completed their time and applied for jobs in government hospitals on their return to civvy street. I informed the family of my decision and after the initial shock horror reaction everyone was soon reconciled to it. I had made a commitment and I was going to honour it and that was that. It wasn't as if I had signed my life away to some dodgy institution.

Moving out of the family house was a real wrench. I had spent so many years in its warm fold. From a young wisp of a lad I had grown into a man within its four walls and become a doctor, the first in the family. There had been good times and bad times and sad times and I had shared them with my grandfather, grandma, father, brothers, sister, friends, relatives. And now I was ready to bid it farewell.

As I was packing my bags with a heavy heart, I recalled the day I heard I had been accepted by the medical college. My father

24

gave me Rs 200 to go to Calcutta with my brother and a cousin and get the medical books I needed for my course. Doubtless Patna was a large city and it had many bookshops, but medical books, well, that was a different matter altogether. I was delighted at the prospect of going to Calcutta. I did my packing – as I was doing now – and a couple of days later we arrived in the bustling city. With our heads in a whirl, we made our way straight for College Street, a truly wonderful, wonderful place with books everywhere – in the shops, stalls, barrows, pavements and wherever the eye went. Oh, what an undiluted thrill it was to be choosing my own books, asking the shopkeeper loudly at times so that everyone present there could know that the subject of my interest was medicine. The books included Gray's *Anatomy*, a voluminous book considered to be the bible of every medical student. It was a pleasant day, a joyous day and soon we had accomplished what we had set out to do.

Just before catching our train back for Patna, my cousin suggested that, as we were all feeling peckish, we should have a bite to eat in a restaurant. The idea was immediately accepted and we headed for an eating place near Howrah Station. We asked for chicken curry and parathas and one or two other things. My brother was not happy with what we had ordered as he was a strict vegetarian and against eating meat in any form or shape. But, being away from home and with no elders watching over us, I let the spirit of adventure take over. In my book of rules, an occasional lapse didn't do any harm. I went ahead with the chicken curry and thoroughly enjoyed my meal.

As we were heading back, I had a sneaky suspicion that my brother wasn't very pleased with what I had done. His looks told me so. We arrived home at night and, exhausted after the long journey, went straight to bed. My worst fears were confirmed in the morning when my brother ratted on me and told grandfather about the chicken curry dinner I had had in Calcutta. All hell broke loose. A Brahmin boy eating chicken and that too in a restaurant – in all probability owned by a Muslim. What was the world coming to! How could I even think of it? In our household such a thing was never done. It was a taboo of the highest order.

My grandfather was simply livid. He stormed into my room and chastised me in the strongest possible terms. I had brought shame on the family. If I did not mend my ways the wrath of all the Hindu gods would get me and so on and so forth. Head-bowed, guilt-ridden, seething inside at my brother for his betrayal, I listened sulkily to everything and accepted that it was entirely my own fault. I had brought it upon myself and should now pay for it. My grandfather despatched me off to the River Ganges where I was to rinse my mouth with its holy water 108 times – same as the number of beads in the Hindu rosary – and then bathe in it in order to atone for my sins. I did what I was told to do as my penance so that I would be allowed back into the house. Forbidden fruit may be sweet, as the proverb goes, but take it from me, forbidden chicken curry can leave a nasty taste in the mouth.

With a suitcase in one hand and a big bag slung over my shoulder, I prepared to head for Lucknow and the headquarters of the Indian Army Medical Corps. I did not know anything about the army or the medical corps but I had made a commitment and I had to keep it. There was, of course, the excitement of the unknown. Frightfully diffident though I may have been, I could not deny that I wanted to be an officer and to wear the uniform of the army. Maybe I was dreaming of seeing the world by being in the medical corps. Maybe I was looking for some excitement in life. There were so many currents and cross-currents running through my head. My brother took me to the railway station and we said our farewell.

The train steamed out of the station and soon the windows were filled with the countryside. We tore through villages and towns with graffiti-scarred backs of houses calling on the British to leave the subcontinent. 'Quit India' demanded the fading words. The click-a-clack rhythm of the train stirred all sorts of memories in my mind and it began to drift back to the time when Mahatma Gandhi's 'Quit India' movement was at its height, generating a lot of nationalistic fervour and anti-British feeling. I was in the fourth year round that time. One afternoon we heard that shots had been fired at protesters in the streets of Patna, resulting in several casualties. As the dead and wounded were brought to our hospital, medical students decided to help in any capacity they could. A number of the students, myself included, took on the role of porters, ferrying the victims of the outrage to the operating theatres and wheeling them out after treatment. Everyone chipped in doing whatever was asked of him. It was a dreadful day. Emotions ran really high. Worried relatives crowded the corridors. Lots of crying, plenty of tears. Angry scenes in the wards. We worked all day and all night, proud that, in our own way, we were doing something for the country and for those who were ready to lay down their lives for it.

I reached Lucknow and reported to the duty officer the next day. I was amazed to find that I wasn't the only one from Patna with hopes and dreams in the heart who had opted to join the army. There were four others from our batch besides me. It was a strange place, Lucknow, full of soldiers bristling in army uniform. Discipline was in the air. You could see it everywhere, in the way those uniformed men greeted each other, in the manner in which they talked, in the stiffness that they displayed in their movement. I wondered what they had for breakfast. Rules and regulations on toast? It was all so alien to me. But a little voice inside told me that, like it or loathe it, I was soon to be a part of it.

That night, a number of us were billeted to the officers' mess. In the morning we collected our kits and our documents. The papers announced I was a lieutenant in the Indian Army Medical Corps. The next three weeks were a real test of endurance. There were around forty in our batch and we had to report to the drilling station each morning. None of us knew much about army drills, but we had to start somewhere. We had drill in the morning, lectures in the afternoon and freedom in the evening. We also had to have a whole series of vaccinations to protect ourselves against a vast range of diseases – malaria, cholera, typhoid, smallpox and plague. The last jab was a really unpleasant one. We knew plague inoculation could cause severe reaction and were not at all looking forward to taking it. One of the lads, Dr Amit Kumar Nath, even made it known to us that he would do everything in his power to avoid it. To the great amazement of everyone in the group he successfully ducked out of it. How he did it only he knew, for he would not reveal it to any of us.

Our training time in Lucknow was soon over and we headed for our next destination, Poona, about a hundred miles from

Bombay. It was a two and a half days' journey by train to Poona. While the slow train wound its way through the hot and dusty plains to the lush green Western Ghats the reaction started, with everyone going down with rigor and high temperature. As we broke into bouts of sweating, we knew what was causing it – except Dr Nath. He was pleased with himself that he had successfully managed to avoid it. Bedraggled, travel-weary and utterly exhausted, we arrived in Poona. I was pleased the journey was finally over, but buried somewhere under the colossal weight of tiredness and the reaction to the plague jab was this little chink of feeling that the first hurdle of our army career was over and we were moving towards the next stage, albeit at a painfully slow pace.

We reported for duty and were put up in tent accommodation. As in Lucknow, we had to undergo six weeks of strict military and medical training. Once again, it was parade in the morning, lectures in the afternoon and free evenings, a routine with which we were so familiar. On the fifth day of training, Dr Nath reported feeling unwell. We were worried about him but we kept our feelings to ourselves. Around that time, a new doctor arrived to join us. Bright, young, intelligent, he seemed a little older than the rest of us. He was also from our medical college in Patna. His name: Kamta Bhargava. I recalled that he was already a house surgeon when we were medical students. Dr Bhargava had made a late decision to join the army and this was the reason he found himself on the same course as us greenhorns. We shared a tent and that was the start of a friendship that lasted until his sad demise in 1992. We remained friends together in India, trained in England in our specialities – he was a surgeon, I a physician. His wife later became a friend of my wife and the friendship then spilled over to the next generation.

While we were attending a military parade one morning the news came that Dr Nath had been admitted to hospital. He was diagnosed to have plague and three days later died of the disease. We were devastated by the news of his death.

The training time in Poona was tedious and, at times, downright unpleasant, but, mercifully, it came to an end after six weeks. However, before that we had to take a written examin-

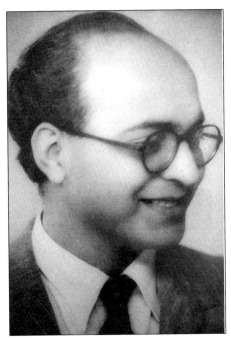

Dr K. P. Bhargava in 1949

ation and an oral test. Besides medicine, they also dealt with military practices. To my utter surprise, I found my name right at the top of the list. Naturally, I was thrilled to bits about my performance in the training, especially on the medical side of it.

With Army training now successfully behind us, it was time to contemplate getting posted somewhere nice and exciting. We spent two or three days wondering what lay ahead, where we would move to, what sort of place it would be. I drew the straw for Deolali. Yes, I was going to Deolali or, to be exact, to work in the military hospital in that place. Reporting for duty, I was surprised to find that I was the only Indian officer there. The rest were British. They were pleasant and courteous but a bit stiff under the collar. We exchanged hellos but nothing more than that. No one ventured beyond the pleasantries and I felt no need to do otherwise. At times it was certainly an ordeal – lots of fidgeting, unease and wondering what was right and what was wrong.

While I was still feeling my way in my job, the colonel of the regiment, quite out of the blue one evening, invited me, the most

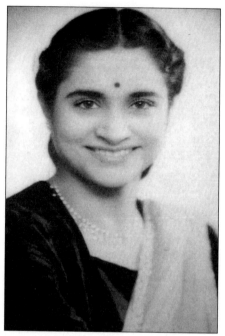

Dr Shanta Bhargava in 1949

junior officer, to his dinner table and to sit next to his wife at the top table. Tightly squeezed into a dinner jacket and with an uneasy grin plastered across my face, I took up my position at the table. Never before had I known that an evening meal could be such a formidable task. For starters, I had to observe all those table manners that I had heard so much about. Then, of course, there was the proper use of knives and forks. How was I going to trap half a dozen peas at the tip of my fork and then bring the fork to my mouth? On top of all this there was the business of having polite conversation with the people on either side of me. The colonel's wife added to my problems by asking how I could toast the King's health with just plain water in my wine glass. But, being a teetotal, I did . . . and with some confidence. The evening passed off without any incident, major or minor. I can't speak for others, but I can honestly say that I was quite pleased with my performance that evening.

With each passing day my confidence grew about being in the army and also about how to deal with people. Being accepted by

British colleagues as an officer helped the process along. But, just as I was settling in nicely, the posting at Deolali came to an end. Orders came that I was to move to Harihar, a town in Mysore state, whose only claim to fame at that time was an army hospital and a regiment stationed there. And, wonder of wonders, I was to be the regimental medical officer.

It was an interesting job because, for the first time in my life, I had to carry out medical inspection of the men in khaki. They stood in a straight line, naked below the waist, to be examined by me. Venereal diseases were quite common at the time and my job was to see if there was any evidence of these men suffering from it. Sure enough, there were a handful with signs of it. These men were asked to report to the medical room the next day. We knew what to do. We had to treat them, make them better, make them fit for their work. The hospital was just a ramshackle of a building but I had drugs, such as penicillin, in plentiful supply.

I stayed in Harihar for six weeks, gained valuable experience in medicine, befriended one or two officers but, on the whole, it wasn't the sort of experience that one pens down in one's diary every night before retiring to bed. Things happened, mostly of a routine nature, some a little out of the ordinary, and that was that. So when the news came that Poona was to be my next stop, I was delighted. There was also talk that it might lead to posting abroad. But before all that I had once again to report to Deolali.

On arrival I heard that the chances of going abroad were minimal but the hospital at Poona would be a new one and it would be under an Indian officer, Colonel J. C. Chandra. The prospect of working in a new hospital was not without its exciting side and it softened some of the disappointment I felt for any chance I had of working abroad slipping through my grasp.

Around twenty-five doctors and other staff were initially needed for posting to the new hospital in Poona. It was to be called 8 Indian British General Hospital (8IBGH). While I waited in Deolali for the official formalities to be completed to move to Poona, my job was to organise and help in the assembling of equipment and other provisions for the proposed hospital. This work had nothing to do with medicine and it provided a pleasant break from medical routine. I would work all day and relax in the evening in the officers' mess with Colonel Chandra and his wife. It was an exciting period because every day one or two new doctors would arrive to join the group for the Poona operation. Meeting new people provided an impetus. Among the new arrivals was Dr Kamta Bhargava. I was pleased to see him and truly happy that we would be together again.

One morning we were summoned to the colonel's office. Colonel Chandra, speaking in a very business-like manner, told us, 'Gentlemen, we're moving to Poona in the next twenty-four hours. You've no hospital. You've no building. We've some tents and we have a job to do. Are you prepared for it? If you think you are, we leave Deolali tomorrow morning.'

Unanimously we said we were ready to take on the job, though we didn't know what the job was and what we were ready for. I suppose the truth was that most of us had no choice in the matter and were making the best of a bad bargain . . . a clear case of when we don't have what we like, we must like what we have.

We, the total workforce plus the paraphernalia we had accumulated in Deolali for the new hospital, arrived in Poona. It was a place I knew well and liked. It was a city with plenty going on and heaps of recreational facilities. I was pleased I was a part of it. Not going abroad did not matter so much now that, like others, I was eager to start work at the new hospital. The day after our arrival in Poona, we were taken to the outskirts of the city where a few animals were grazing peacefully in a field. There were a couple of sheds near which about half a dozen tents were pitched. It looked like the site for a small farm show. We were flabbergasted when someone announced that this was our hospital. Although we were aware that we were heading for the unknown, this was just too much. We looked at each other dejectedly, then at the sheds and tents and the cows who, to add insult to our injury, mooed loudly. We shook our heads with sheer disbelief. Silently, I asked myself if this was what I had volunteered to join the army for. Similar thoughts were going through the minds of my colleagues, I learned later. The only ray of hope in all this chaotic mess was that we had good friends and talking about our problems to each other, if it did not make them disappear, it at least reduced their size.

The next two years in Poona had their exciting moments. We were promised the tented hospital would soon be replaced with one in a first-rate building. There would be proper wards for patients, well-equipped operating theatres and what have you. Within a short period, temporary accommodation was created and we occupied parts of the buildings from an older hospital nearby, which was basically a military hospital for patients arriving from the Far East. I soon realised that the new hospital would deal mainly with tuberculosis, because soldiers who came to India from that part of the world suffered mainly from TB – pulmonary, hip or spine.

One evening we were summoned and told to have plaster beds ready for a group of six patients arriving from the Far East. By now the staff number had grown considerably and included several British doctors and nurses. They were friendly and a delight to work with and we got on marvellously well. One of the nurses, Sister George, who had done her training in Edinburgh, was allocated to our team. She was attractive, lively, competent and a good team player. If you were down in the dumps or suffering from a bout of low morale, Sister George was just the person. A simple chat with her acted like a tonic.

We set about our task of preparing the beds. Next morning, a fleet of ambulances arrived carrying twenty patients, all suffering, all needing urgent attention, all desperate for a plaster bed. Then there were other patients who needed plaster casts. All told there were sixty of them. Six of us, two doctors, two nurses and two orderlies, worked like people possessed throughout the night and by daybreak had casts for all of them. Then, through sheer exhaustion, we collapsed.

Two English surgeons, Major Jack Collis and Major H. Muller, were very impressed with our effort. Major Collis – he later became Colonel Collis – thought it was a tremendous achievement, worthy of a prize. To look after the TB sufferers a team was formed comprising a sister, an orderly and myself. Taking care of them was a hard and physically demanding job. The patients were immobile in plaster casts, and, it being a new hospital, we had no experience to fall back upon. As the number of patients admitted to 8IBGH increased, it soon became a major hospital and was taken up by the Indian Government. The intention was to turn it into a leading centre for chest treatment. I was privileged to be a part of it.

Major Collis was a very competent doctor. He was kind and helpful and we soon became friends. He was an inspiration to me. Once again the friendship lasted a lifetime, until his death in Britain. I attended his memorial service to pay tribute to him. He had taught me medicine in the army and told me I was capable of greater things and, if I decided to come to Britain to get postgraduate qualifications, I could stay with him until I found my feet. When I did come to Britain I got in touch with him and he introduced me to the medical fraternity in Birmingham. Our friendship went beyond the two of us; I was particularly fond of his children.

One day in the Poona hospital Major Collis came to see me and said that he was going to see a private patient and asked me if I could help him out in the operating theatre. Frankly, I felt flattered to have been asked. Little did I know that 'helping out in the operating theatre' entailed assisting in a surgical operation and at that time I had limited experience in that field. Next morning I went with him to the hospital where the operation was to take place. The patient was Lady Brabourne, a relative of the Governor of Bombay. She had fallen off a horse and cracked a rib and sustained other injuries. We entered the operating theatre and, after going through the pre-operational routine, took our position, ready for surgery on the patient lying on the operating table.

It transpired then that the table was a bit high for me to assist Major Collis in the operation. The sister helping us was an extremely resourceful person. To make me taller for the job in hand she whizzed off to her office and returned with a couple of drawers from her office cupboard. With a triumphant smile she turned them upside down and her open palm instructed me to step on them. Eureka! I had gained eight inches in height, possibly more, in the twinkling of an eye. What a morale booster that was! The operation started and was proceeding smoothly when I began to experience a funny sensation underneath my feet. The wood was cracking and I was slowly losing height, coming down to earth from my exalted position. In a panic I shouted, 'Sister, I'm going through your drawers.' There was total silence for a moment. Major Collis brought it to an end by saying, 'Really, Dr Chatterjee?'

If the earth had opened up before me at that moment I would've gladly dived into the hole to hide my embarrassment. The whole operating unit burst into a boisterous laugh. The operation was as successful as the goings-on in the theatre were hilarious. It marked another important point in my military career, for I had never come across a situation like that before.

CHAPTER 4

Days of decision

THE HOSPITAL IN POONA was in its formative years. I was
fortunate to be a part of its medical team at this exciting stage
of its development, as it was later to become one of the leading
tuberculosis and chest hospitals in the country. The doctors who
worked in it were from both Britain and India. They were all
well-qualified, well-experienced and dedicated people. Most of
them, myself included, lived in Aundh, about six miles away.

I was elected, much against my wishes, as the wine officer in
the officers' mess. It was an important position. It made me in
charge of every drink that was served to the officers who, after a
hard day's slog, took their relaxation pretty seriously and so the
margin for error was quite slim. Just a few days into the job, I saw
an opportunity to raise extra revenue for the officers' mess. I
proposed that the price of every drink be raised by two rupees.
The hike was agreed by the management committee and in just
six months we had made profit that was described as 'more than
handsome'. My colleagues were very happy with the extra money
raised, as it considerably reduced their share of the cost of running
the mess and keeping the living accommodation in good shape.

In the hospital, I was in charge of two medical wards with a
team comprising another medical officer, Dr Gerald Crocket, a
sister and a nurse. Dr Crocket was an anaesthetist but he also
helped in the day-to-day running of the wards. The two of us got
on marvellously well, became friends and remained so all the time
we were in 8IBGH and even later. When I came to Britain I met
him several times in Northampton and we raised glasses to each
other.

One of my duties in the early days at 8IBGH was to escort
army personnel who were on the move from and to various parts
of the country. Our quartermaster was Major Tiny Rowland, a
big bulk of a human being, kind, generous and full of laughs and
jokes. This gentle giant was a non-medical officer and a bundle

of fun to be with. He knew I was from the eastern part of the country and whenever he had soldiers to escort to that region he would ask me if I was interested to go home. I would leap at the chance. I would then take on the role of the regimental medical officer for a few weeks from Poona to the eastern region. This was roughly a three-day rail journey with many longish stops on the way.

There were usually around 2,000 men in khaki on the train and the medical officer was in charge of their physical well-being during the trip. Normally these journeys posed no major problems. On reaching Patna, I would rush to our place for three or four days of home comforts, including ample rest and hot, straight-from-the-kitchen meals, before setting off for Poona for the return journey. I would classify these trips as the enjoyable part of army life.

Meanwhile the learning process continued apace. Colonel Collis – he had now been promoted from the rank of major – was in charge of our division. He taught me a lot about medicine and plenty about surgery and I was often complimented by him for the work I was doing in my wards. In moments of relaxation I would discuss with him my plans for the future. He would listen attentively, absorb all that I said, but he would not comment. One day, over a cup of tea, I told him I was tinkering with the idea of studying for a postgraduate degree. He agreed that it was necessary if I wanted to progress in my field. Then, out of the blue, he fixed his gaze on me and asked, 'Would you like to go to England for your postgrad degree?'

Going abroad was something I had given thought to in the past, but every time an opportunity came along it was quickly snuffed out by one thing or another, mainly the demands of the job in the Army. I was aware that most of the doctors in important positions in our medical college in Patna, such as professors and senior lecturers, had been to England for higher qualifications. I had also on more occasions than one entertained the idea of becoming a member of the Royal College of Physicians. After all, it was the coveted prize if you wanted to make headway in your profession.

'Is it hard work, studying for a postgrad degree in England?' I asked Colonel Collis somewhat naively.

'Oh, it certainly is,' he said. 'I'm a surgeon and not a physician so I can't really tell you how hard, but it is hard.'

'I thought so.'

'But should you decide to go ahead with the idea and proceed to England, you can stay with me for a few days to get yourself acquainted with the system.'

'Of course I will. Course!' I stammered, unable to contain myself. I didn't expect that kind of offer from anybody, but coming from my own English officer, it sounded just unbelievable. To this day I'm indebted to Colonel Collis – he became Professor Collis on his return to England – for his help and guidance. He pointed the direction to me and then made sure that I had covered the first mile.

In free time at 8IBGH, we either went fell walking in the hills around Poona or strolled in the mountains on the beautiful, lush green Western Ghats, scene of many fiercely fought battles between the invading Muslims and the local Maratha warriors. But we rarely ventured further afield. However, a team of officers once planning a trip to the historic city of Aurangabad to see the Ajanta and Ellora caves, nearly 400 miles from Poona, asked me if I would like to join them. The organiser of this expedition was Colonel Satish Bannerjee. Being single, I was a bit reluctant when I heard that some of the officers were also taking their wives and children with them. But on Colonel Bannerjee's insistence I gave in. A few days later, one morning at the crack of dawn, the party set off in four cars. It was a long journey by the standards prevailing at the time, travel conditions being what they were.

After some sightseeing on the way we arrived at the caves which are at different locations. Nearly 2,000 years of artistic activity is recorded in a series of rock-cut caves at Ajanta and Ellora as well as the Buddhist caves at Aurangabad. The caves were temples and monasteries around 400 AD. There are stone-carvings as well as paintings of figures from Indian mythology. In fact, the world's largest monolithic monument is there in the shape of a royal temple complex, with elaborate sculptures everywhere. Even today they are a huge tourist attraction and a testimony to what wonders man is capable of with a simple chisel, a hammer and imagination. We stayed in a bungalow at Ajanta, explored the caves at night and moved on to Ellora the next morning. It was truly one of the most remarkable and interesting holidays I've ever had in my life. To this day I vividly remember some of the figures I saw in those caves. Apart from the caves, there were plenty of other minor attractions in the area, such as waterfalls, wildlife and birds.

Back from the holiday, I decided to pursue my plan to go to England for further studies. I wanted to learn more about medicine and a degree from Blighty was good for the profession I had chosen. I had, in the meantime, received an invitation from Delhi to attend an interview for a permanent commission in the Army. Although a voice inside told me that the future lay in obtaining a postgraduate degree from England, followed by a stint of work there to gain some experience, I decided, half-heartedly, to attend the interview.

Perhaps it was this lukewarm approach that led to my poor showing in the interview. On my return from Delhi I learned that I had been unsuccessful. This stiffened my resolve to quit the Army. From then on it was a case of just carrying on until the right moment arrived. The next few months went by doing the usual routine things – work, studies, managing the mess. There were also the usual outings with fellow officers, nurses and other members of staff. Towards the end of 1946, I officially applied to leave the Army. We celebrated Christmas and the New Year with great enthusiasm. Colonel Chandra looked after us very well. During the festive period he asked me about my plans and I told him I was planning to go to England for further studies.

'It's a jolly good idea, but how would you go?' he demanded.

'By boat, of course,' I replied.

'I can guess that, but there're a hell of a number of other things you have to do first before you can set foot on the boat.' Colonel Chandra then gave me a litany of documents I needed before I could begin the journey. I had to get a passport and that meant finding a guarantor. Then there was the matter of a ticket for the ship, injections against diseases, income tax clearance and heaven knows what else. The upshot of all this was that I became terribly disheartened with the whole project. Why was life so damned complicated?

A couple of days later, I received a telephone call in my ward. Colonel Chandra wanted me to see him in his office. Normally, if he wanted to see a junior officer in his office it spelt trouble for that officer. Naturally, I was worried. With great trepidation, I went to see him and waited outside his office for a few moments to compose myself. I knocked on the door, went in and saluted him.

'Take a seat.' He pointed to a chair.

'Thank you, sir. You wanted to see me?'

'Oh yes. You want to go to England?' he inquired.

'Yes, sir. I think I told you the other day.'

'You remember I said something about a guarantor that you'd need to sponsor you?'

'Yes, sir. I do.'

'Well, I've decided that I'll be your guarantor. I'll sign your passport form. Just bring it to me after you've filled it in.'

'Thank you, sir.'

'Or better still, I'll get you a passport form. You just fill it in. I'll also give you the name and address of a person who works in Bombay Secretariat. Go and see him and he'll get you the passport.'

I saluted him, much more stiffly to show my gratitude, and came out of his office with my head on cloud nine and my imagination floating in the mists of outer space. What a welcome situation it was! It was common knowledge among most Indians that getting a passport entailed a wait of at least six months because of all the red tape involved and here was my own officer offering to arrange it for me in days I could count on the fingers of my hands.

I went to Bombay and headed straight for the secretariat where this angel of a man held an important position and was going to work wonders for me. He gave a look which could hardly be called friendly and shifted his glance to the form and the various attachments it carried, went through the lot thoroughly, carefully, occasionally giving me a surreptitious look. This went on for a long time, my heart thumping loudly in case he found something wanting in the papers. The scrutiny over, he said to me, 'Come back in three hours and collect your passport.' I thanked him profusely and left to while away three hours, giving myself a small treat in one of Bombay's myriad Irani restaurants. When I returned, true to his word, he had the passport in front of him signed, stamped and endorsed. He handed it to me without ceremony. I was ecstatic with joy. I felt like doing a hand walk for the man to show my appreciation for what he had done for me.

I returned to Poona in a triumphal mood and quickly settled down into the old routine, but now my mind was elsewhere. I had already served more than two and a half years in the Army and learned most of what I thought it could teach me. By this time, British Army officers were being demobbed and planning to return home.

'I take it you're going to England?' Colonel Collis asked me one evening after work.

'Yes, sir,' I replied, joyfully.

'Can you do me a favour?' he asked.

'Sure, fire away,' I answered, remembering the number of favours he had done to me.

'I have two trunks, one full of medical equipment and the other containing curtain material and some items of clothing. Would you be kind enough to bring them with you? You're, of course, coming to stay with us for a few days, aren't you?'

'Of course I am. The trunks will be no problem.'

It wasn't just the British officers who were leaving the hospital. The Indians were also on the move. The team, forged together over a number of months, was now breaking up. Colonel Chandra was promoted to brigadier and transferred. His replacement was Colonel Rao, a tall man, rather aloof, who, it came as no surprise, was more interested in people who were staying on than those who were going. He called me into his office and broke the news that my demob papers had arrived and I was free to leave in the next three months. He had also made the necessary arrangements with the accounts people to have my gratuity and other payments worked out in time for my departure. This was important because I was depending on this money to pay for my passage to England. Another piece had fallen into place in my scheme of things.

My papers arrived and I completed the official formalities of leaving. I was ready for civilian life once more. I was pleased that before long I'd be back in Patna and there would be long and lazy days of rest and inactivity after the homecoming. It was a time of mixed feelings. India had been promised independence by Britain. On the one hand I was happy India was going to be a free country in a few months' time, ready to chart its own future, but on the other hand I was sad that, I was going to lose so many colleagues with whom I had forged a bond that went well beyond the everyday calls of duty. In April 1947, I went to Bombay again and arranged with a shipping line for my passage to England. The arrangement was a tentative one. Final booking and payments were to follow later.

The two-day journey to Patna was full of memories of the three years I had spent in the Army. Coloured by time and nostalgia, every experience as a uniformed officer now seemed pleasant. The countryside whizzing by on the outside and my head leaning against the train window on the inside, I recalled how, in extremely adverse conditions, doctors and nurses, both British and Indian, and the Indian ancillary staff, had battled against the odds to save the lives of fighting men. The excellent team spirit they had built up and displayed in their everyday work was a lesson, certainly to me. During those years I had changed from a scraggy, bashful fellow to a competent and confident officer perfectly capable of dealing with life at any level. The discipline and the regimental ways, which I so detested at times, suddenly seemed to have served me well. Out of the Army now, I was glad I had been a part of it for three years.

When I arrived in Patna my brother, who had always been more like a friend than a brother, was there at the railway station to meet me. We went home, talking all the time like two little schoolboys on the way, mostly about what had happened in my life in the past few days. I went into my room and stayed there for a long time, thinking. The scene at home had changed. My sister-in-law was now firmly established as the matron of the house. She was also the mother of a little girl whom they had named Stella and who had been born just a few months earlier.

Although I was home now, I felt terribly lonely because I had no close friends and the medical fraternity in the city was alien to me. I arranged to meet one or two doctors to find out about job prospects. I also went back to the medical college and was told I could join as a houseman, but the offer, if offer it could be called, somehow did not appeal to me. Out of nowhere a conflict had arisen in my mind. I wanted to go to England while at the same time I was looking for job opportunities in India.

One or two people suggested that I should take up the job at the medical college and then apply for leave to go overseas for further studies. But this approach was fraught with complexities and entailed giving all manner of undertakings and treading the uncharted path of medical politics. It was all very confusing and added to my dithering. My father had just retired from his government job and wasn't much help in the matter when I sought his advice. 'The final decision is yours' was his mantra, his wise words, every time I raised the subject. However, one of his friends, a round-faced, pleasant man who mostly wore a starched, white *dhoti* and *kurta*, proved helpful in a strange sort of way when I put my quandary to him.

'I can't make up my mind but I think I'd like to go to England and do my membership of the Royal College of Physicians,' I said to him when he came for tea to our house one evening. 'I don't know a single soul in that country and all I have is an offer by a former colleague and friend of a few days' accommodation in his house.'

He nodded his head sagely, indicating he was beginning to understand my dilemma.

'I've to apply for jobs, meet new people who can guide me, help me. I'd also like to work there, make a living while I prepare for my exams.'

All of a sudden, as if by magic, the expression on his face changed. With a look of total amazement, he said, 'What are you worried about?'

'Just that I don't know whether it's the right thing or not?'

He took a longish sip of tea from his Bengal Pottery cup, seemed to think for a while, nodding his head all the time, and then asked me to bring two pieces of string, of different colours. I obeyed, left the room and returned with a white string and a red one. As I extended my hand with the strings in his direction he asked me to choose one of the two. I didn't know what to make of it. Nonetheless I picked the red string with the other hand.

'See,' he said with a degree of enthusiasm, 'you didn't know which one to pick, did you? You could've picked the other one but you didn't.'

This string game left me utterly baffled. 'What do you mean?' I asked politely.

'It's all very simple. You've two choices: go to England and study further or stay in India, get a job, marry, settle down and all the rest. Am I right?'

'Of course, you are.'

'You chose the former. You could've chosen the latter, but you didn't. Once you've made the choice, have no regrets. Follow the choice you've made wholeheartedly. If at some stage in the future you feel you've made the wrong choice, just consider it a piece of tough luck but remember it was the right choice at the time you made it.'

I studied his face for a moment and felt a little reassured. Looking back, I can say with all honesty that I made the right choice then. After that meeting I made up my mind that I'd accept the offer from the shipping line of the first available place on the boat for England. But there was one problem: I had no money. Well, not enough to pay for the passage and have some to see me through the first few days in the new country. Whatever I had earned in the past three years I had spent in the past three years, most of it at any rate, except the gratuity which I had received only on leaving the Army.

When I told my father about it, he called me into his room for a little heart-to-heart and said, 'Look, son, I can't give you an awful lot of money, simply because I haven't got it, but here's a cheque from me to you. Take it with my blessings.' He folded a piece of paper and handed it to me. I accepted it, without looking at it, and touched his feet, as is customary in most Indian households when you receive a gift from an elder. My eyes were moist with infant tears at his concern for me. A few minutes later I unfolded the cheque and, to my utter amazement, found that it was for Rs 10,000 – a small fortune in old money and enough to keep me going for over a year in England. I was deeply moved. Here was my father, who had kept his emotions bottled up most of his life, now old, retired, in poor health, giving me a big chunk of his savings to ensure I was all right, at least in the money department, in the new and faraway land I had chosen to go to.

About a week later a letter arrived from the shipping line offering me a berth on the SS *Strathmore* which was leaving from Bombay on 12 May 1947. I readily accepted the offer and sent the money. My documents were in order and I had taken all the necessary jabs while in the Army. However, I needed new shoes and some warm clothes for the English winters. I had an overcoat from the Army but, being khaki, it was of little use in civilian life. So, instead of getting a new one, I had it dyed black. Problem solved!

In a matter of days I was ready to set off. A big party was organised for me at home. Lots of friends and relatives came to wish me luck in my endeavour. But amid the jolly atmosphere of the party I detected a certain sadness in my father's eyes. Even at that late stage, he didn't want me to leave home. I snatched moments of privacy in my own room to feel sad myself. A son – and a doctor son at that – is like a promissory note that matures in your old age. Throughout your life you pay premiums in the form of providing good education, decent clothes, a good upbringing. But now that it was time for him to cash that promissory note, his son was waving a goodbye. And then there was the emotional side.

Early in May, on a warm night, I said farewell to my father. Outside the house, there was a *tonga* waiting to take me to Patna railway station, the horse in the cart neighing a sort of time reminder. My father ran his hand over my head and gave his final blessing. 'Do come back, will you?' he mumbled, in a voice choking with emotion. I promised I would, more with gestures than with voice, because deep inside I knew it wouldn't be for a long time. We exchanged a look and I experienced this feeling that it was my final goodbye to him. I never saw him again. He died before I could go back.

My brother came with me to the station and then carried on with me on the train to Gaya, where I was to change for the overnight express to Bombay. I stayed one night in a hotel close to the docks and next day went with my luggage to Ballard Pier where the SS *Strathmore* was berthed. After the official formalities were over and the departure time for the ship was approaching, I stepped on the gangway, mentally raised a celebratory fist and yelled, 'England, here I come!'

CHAPTER 5

The great adventure

UNDER A CLEAR, blue sky, with not a single cloud in sight, the USS *Strathmore* majestically set sail for England. Hundreds of passengers stood at various levels to bid farewell to Bombay and watched the ship gently pull away from the dock. I waved frantically, to no one particular, my mind filled with a heady cocktail of excitement and anxiety – almost in equal measure – and it was making me giddy.

I was excited because my great adventure had finally begun and anxious because I didn't know what lay ahead once the journey was over in a fortnight. How hard would the exams for the Membership of the Royal College of Physicians be? Would I be the right person in the right place once I had qualified? Would the playing fields be level when looking for a job? If not, how would I cope? Questions crowded my mind.

The SS *Strathmore* was a huge ship which had been used during the war for transporting soldiers. At the time of our travel, it had still not been fully refurbished to civilian standards. We were put in the big hold right at the bottom of the ship, with plenty of space and hammock-like beds. Cleanliness was well up to standard and the food was plentiful and quite enjoyable. There was Indian food, Continental cuisine and English delicacies on the menu – something to suit every palate. The ship had nearly 1,500 people on board – a handful of Europeans, but mostly Indians and Anglo-Indians. Some were going to England for business, others for further studies, many for work.

As the journey got under way and the ship picked up speed, the passengers relaxed and began to mix and mingle. Within no time I found myself a part of an eight-strong group. We moved together, had our meals together and discussed our future as it was the main focus of our attention and concentrated our minds. It was then I discovered that I wasn't the only one with a few butterflies fluttering in the stomach. Most of us were ordinary, decent fellows, with a good education and from stable back-grounds who had led well-organised, orderly lives in which the family had played an important part and for whom sound economic health not only mattered but was in a way essential. But now, sailing on the high seas, we were without the family's safety net and an economic base was just a holy grail whose search had barely begun. We had to make something of ourselves – by ourselves. We could not look up to anyone for help. All the help lay at the end of our own arms.

I also had my medical text books with me and whatever free time I had I devoted to them, reading a little each day. There were plenty of things going on all the time on the boat and in the sea around us on all sides. It was indeed a thrill watching the flying fish doing their acrobatics in the water and the Arab dhows battling with the waves, carrying grain to various destinations. There were also a number of other small boats engaged in their own business.

We passed Aden and entered the Red Sea. The sun was searingly hot, but it didn't seem to affect us, because we had dreams in our hearts and adventure on our minds. My knowledge about England was at best sketchy, maybe marginally better, but I was fired up by the desire to study further, gain valuable experience and become important, something of a role model. I had enough resources to see me through for up to two years if I kept a watchful eye on my expenditure. So, as far as the money side was concerned, I was all right. In an ideal world I would have liked an attachment, paid or unpaid, to a medical unit, so that I could study cases, use the unit's facilities and fast-forward my learning. As I saw it then it was the best way forward, the practical way to become a better doctor. But sadly such an ideal world existed only in my own imagination. No doubt reality would unfold soon enough and tell an altogether different tale.

The Red Sea was dull and terribly humid and rumours abounded on board that even the most experienced sailors found it insufferable. But, surprisingly, the ship sailed through it without any major problem and we soon found ourselves in the Suez Canal, just a strip of water, man-made and narrow, so narrow, in fact, that you could almost touch both sides of land from the ship, Egypt on one side, Arabia on the other.

At Port Suez we stopped for a few hours and then entered the Mediterranean, which was at first calm and peaceful. Everyone in our group talked a lot about England and the English way of life, our pool of knowledge about the new country increasing every hour. Someone in our group enlightened us that the English landladies were formidable creatures if you failed to pay your rent on the nail, friendly and pleasant if you handed over the cash on time and downright charming if you paid in advance. He had heard this from someone who had heard it from someone else.

In the Bay of Biscay the ship was pounded by mountainous waves. The sea was in full fury and the sky above was almost black with rain clouds. The SS *Strathmore* was no more than a cork floating in a mighty ocean, battered from all sides. It felt as if we were part of a scene from some sea disaster movie. The experience was utterly frightening and nearly all of us were seasick, homesick, tired and torn with anxiety. There was a huge collective sigh of relief when it was announced that the ship would soon be arriving at Southampton. We were still absorbing the knowledge that our journey was about to come to an end when a further announcement brought new problems. The voice on the public address system told us that porters at Southampton were on strike and that we would have to take care of our own baggage. Apart from my own paraphernalia, I was also carrying two large cases for Mr Collis.

The morning was dull and grey, with a fine drizzle, when the ship reached Southampton on 24 May 1947. We had our documents checked by immigration officials and by the time the formalities were over it was nearly midday. We were now free to go wherever we wanted. Although I was now in England, I still had some distance to go to reach my final destination. I had to catch a train from Southampton to London and from there another one for Birmingham. At a rough guess a day's journey lay ahead of me. I telephoned the Collis household to announce my arrival in the country but could not give a definite time of arrival in Birmingham because I did not know myself when I would reach the Midlands and the security of the Collis household.

The train journey from Southampton to London was truly an experience. I kept my eyes open and observed people, lots of

people, doing lots of things. They were quiet but helpful,
courteous to each other, opening doors, holdings doors for others,
saying 'thank you' at the slightest pretext and 'sorry' for reasons I
couldn't work out, but in the main minding their own business,
mostly reading paperbacks and newspapers. This observer role can
be very fascinating, especially on your very first day in a new
country when your powers of observation are at their sharpest.
Everything is a change for the system and these first images and
impressions remain with you for a long time. Anyway, fascinating
or not, it certainly kept my mind occupied. By the time I reached
Euston, after a train journey and a taxi ride, it was evening and
Birmingham was still nowhere in sight. My guess was that it lay
about a hundred miles away. But time passed as it always does and
I completed the final leg of my long haul at about 11p.m. Yes,
finally I found myself at Birmingham New Street but felt a few
shivers run down my spine because it was cold at that time of the
night. Light rain was also falling so I decided not to go to Mr
Collis's house and spent the night at the railway station.

For a stranger just arrived, Birmingham New Street at that
hour was an unfriendly place. There was no sleeping accommodation at the station for passengers who, for one reason or
another, found themselves forced to spend the night there. There
was a small waiting room in which a group of people were
crammed together, with only a small heater in the wall to keep
them warm. I insinuated myself into that group but sleep was
obviously out of the question, though some people kept dozing
on and off until it was morning.

As the day broke, I splashed some cold water – that was the
only variety available – on my face, dragged myself to the taxi
stand, threw myself into a taxi and instructed the driver to take
me to Harbourne Road where Mr Collis lived with his family.
When I got out, a pleasant surprise greeted me. At the door of
the house Mrs Collis was waiting with her two children, one at
each side. I had barely wished her the time of day when she
demanded, 'Where have you been, Dr Chatterjee? We waited all
night for you. We've been worried sick in case . . .'

I was dumbfounded. A warm handshake with her and the
smiles of the children told me I was home – away from home. I

apologised two or three times and explained that I did not want to disturb the family at that late hour. 'Disturb? Nonsense. You're our guest. You're going to be with us for a few days. I hope you like it here.' Feeling truly welcomed, I looked at her gratefully and thanked Mrs Collis. 'Don't call me Mrs Collis, please. Just Mavis.' And for the next few days Mavis was my guardian angel, showing me around, explaining things to me, answering my myriad queries. I felt lucky I had come to Birmingham.

That afternoon Mr Collis came home from the hospital and we had a long chat about what I was to do and how I was to do it. He reiterated that I was welcome to stay with the family for as long as I liked. I thanked him in return and reassured him that I'd move out as soon as I could see the way ahead clear. Next morning he took me to his place of work, the Queen Elizabeth Hospital. It was a large teaching hospital where a lot of doctors prepared for further qualifications in various specialities. Mr Collis was a professor now. I had only MBBS to my name, which was just a basic medical degree. I was single-minded about adding postgraduate qualifications to it as quickly as circumstances allowed. Mr Collis introduced me to a number of doctors and other members of his staff. I told them I wasn't looking for a job, merely a chance to be present as an observer when outpatients and some inpatients were being examined.

My first few days in Birmingham were very pleasant, though not without a degree of anxiety. Mr Collis told me he would set up meetings with a couple of general practitioners so that I could have more varied experience of the system and widen my net when it came to looking for a job. One of the people I met at the hospital was Dr Clifford Hawkins, a consultant in one of the medical units. He offered to take me under his wing. The arrangement was that he would instruct and guide me on how to put my plans into operation – for a small charge. There were several other doctors with their own plans who were also ready to join his group.

My stay with the Collis family was a comfortable one. I had a room to myself where I could study without any disturbance. Then there were home-cooked meals and, above all, a pleasant and supportive family with whom I could share my free time and keep loneliness at bay. A few days went by and I asked Mavis how much I owed her.

'Owe what?' Her face was a picture of amazement. 'You owe me nothing. Don't even think about it. You're a friend of the family.'

Strange, I thought to myself, we were never told about this brand of landlady on the ship. A couple of days later she announced that an outing had been planned: we were all going to see a play. I was really pleased to hear that as it had been a few days since I had been out. The first play that I saw in Britain was Oscar Wilde's *Lady Windermere's Fan*.

One day while I was attending an outpatient clinic, one of the doctors, Professor Melville Arnott, told me about a GP in Great Barr, north Birmingham, by the name of Dr Hiren Roy. He suggested that it would be worthwhile meeting him. At the first available opportunity I took a bus from Edgbaston and made my way to see Dr Roy. Great Barr was a quiet district of Birmingham with a lot of neat houses on leafy roads. At the corner of one such road was his surgery. I knocked on the door and there in front of me stood the smiling figure of Dr Roy. He welcomed me in after a warm handshake. 'I've heard a lot about you,' said the GP in a pleasant, courteous voice.

'Same here,' I answered, happy in the knowledge that a Bengali doctor like me had successfully established himself in England and was a medic to be emulated. The pleasantries soon over, Dr Roy told me he had no position to offer me but if I helped him in his work from time to time there would be some financial compensation for my endeavours, though not a lot. I agreed. The arrangement suited me well. I did not want a busy, full-time job until I had done my membership exam. I also made it clear to Dr Roy that my main objective was to do hospital medicine.

We met again the same evening, this time for a meal. Also joining us was his wife. We talked at length on many subjects, mainly to do with medicine. At some point during the evening he suggested that I should move to Great Barr and that he would help me in the hunt for digs. Being close to the surgery would greatly reduce time spent on travelling. I was pleased things were going according to plan. Satisfied, I went back to Edgbaston and told Mr Collis about doing sessions in Dr Roy's surgery.

Two or three days later, on a bright Sunday morning, Mr and Mrs Collis took me in their car to my new place in Great Barr and I was installed in my digs. Once again I had a room to myself but this time breakfast and evening meals were included in the deal and money had a role to play in the arrangement. The total weekly cost of all this in old money was £2. 10s. The new place suited me well as it was within walking distance of a bus stop from where I could take public transport to the Queen Elizabeth Hospital after the morning surgery at Dr Roy's and back again in time for the evening clinic, although the latter was more off than on. While attending the outpatients' department in the hospital I came into regular contact with two consultants – Dr Oscar Brenner, a cardiologist who was a well-known and highly-respected figure in his field and, of course, Dr Hawkins. Both of them told me I could see their patients on one-day-a-week basis.

So for the next eight months I attended Dr Roy's surgery in the morning, saw outpatients in the hospital in the early afternoon and then spent the later part of the day in the hospital library studying in greater detail cases I had earlier dealt with and also preparing for my membership exam. At the same time I was taking instructions from Dr Hawkins on patient diagnosis, clinical lectures, writing and how to prepare for the exams. After these eight months of guidance from him I felt a lot more confident and thought I was ready for the test.

During a session at his surgery, Dr Roy introduced me to a man, tall, dignified but terribly short of breath. He worked as an assistant telephone manager and was at the time suffering from acute bronchitis. 'This is Dr Chatterjee' said Dr Roy, by way of introduction. 'He's an expert in the illness you're suffering from.' He shifted his gaze to the patient and added, 'This is Mr Joseph Adlington.'

We shook hands with polite formality.

'Would you help me?' the patient asked, in a low voice.

I nodded affirmatively. He seemed a sort of father figure to me. 'I'll definitely try.'

Little did I know then that, in the days and years to come, my life would be inextricably linked to the Adlington family. A few days later I visited the family house and was introduced to a pleasant young woman, Miss Enid Adlington, who, like her father, worked at the telephone office. We soon became friends. She was kind, affectionate, and genuinely interested in my plans. In December that year I received a Christmas card from Miss Adlington and an invitation from the family to spend Christmas with them. The Adlington hospitality was overwhelming. The couple were generous, friendly, and kind. From friends, Miss Adlington and I became good friends.

The day of the membership exam of the Royal College of Physicians was fast approaching but my preparation for it was by no means complete. However, March 1948 soon arrived and I headed for London for the big test. In those days there was just one exam stretched over three weeks in four stages. On the first day it was pen to paper all the time – endless words scribbled in a hurry. Thoughts, facts and figures poured out with quick-fire rapidity. At the end of it all, I thought I hadn't done as well as I should have. But to my great surprise I sailed through the clinical as well as the written parts. Pathology and the viva were the next hurdles, followed by a final oral test.

It's always difficult to sit in judgement of yourself, especially in matters as tricky as exams. When you fear you've done badly, the examiner may find you were up to the mark and when you feel you were all right, he or she may have different ideas. That was the case with the viva and pathology. Things were proceeding satisfactorily as far as I was concerned, but soon I began to detect an approach of superior indifference creeping in towards the young candidates who had come for the exam. Some of the examiners seemed more critical of the way the presentation was made than of the presentation itself. The doughnut was being judged by the roundness of the hole. Shadow appeared more important than substance.

The next day I received a letter telling me that I had not been successful. Naturally, I was terribly disappointed. Back in Birmingham I told Miss Adlington about it. She showed a lot of understanding and was very supportive and sympathetic. She said that I'd have to work a lot harder the next time. The next time she was talking about arrived a month later. It was the same routine all over again – and unfortunately the same result. But each setback only stiffened my resolve. Victory was mine in the end and I became a Member of the Royal College of Physicians. So overjoyed was I that, on the day I learned that, I wanted to tell the whole world about it from every rooftop in London. But there was only one person I knew in the great metropolis: Dr Sunil Bhattacharya, once a fellow student with me back in Patna. He had also made his way to England and was now working in a surgery in London. He had been a constant source of encouragement to me. We met at Pall Mall and a celebration ensued.

I returned to Birmingham, my head in the yonder reaches of outer space, and proceeded to meet Miss Adlington and break the news. Almost tap dancing with excitement, in one breath I told her about my success and with the next proposed to her. Inside me I knew all along she was the perfect partner for me. And how time has proved me right. For more than fifty years she has been a true soulmate. Words of love, nudges of encouragement, offers of help spoken and unspoken – I've had them all from her and a lot more besides, things that make life a long, wonderful experience. I was lucky!

With MRCP under my belt, I was now ready to launch myself as a professional into the world of medicine in England. Within no time I had three interviews lined up – in Birmingham, Manchester and Newcastle upon Tyne. After some deliberation and consultation, I plumped for the Walker Gate Hospital in Newcastle. Enid was with me when I went in for my interview. She wished me luck and began her anxious countdown. When I came out I was a registrar in thoracic medicine.

17 July 1949 was a memorable day. I was studying something in the library in Birmingham when a doctor telephoned to congratulate me on becoming a father. My wife had just given birth to a baby girl. Thrilled to bits, I rushed to the maternity ward of the hospital to see Enid and the new addition to the family. Picking up the little bundle of joy I muttered, 'Welcome, Camille.' Or words to that effect.

Within just over two years of arriving in Britain some of the most important things in my life had happened to me: I had become a Member of the Royal College of Physicians; I had also become a husband and a father; and I had found a job in a hospital. I had, at least by my own reckoning, come a long way.

CHAPTER 6

Newcastle and Manchester

WHEN I OPTED FOR NEWCASTLE, the thinking behind the preference was that the Walker Gate Hospital in the city was smaller than those in Birmingham and Manchester and therefore it was an ideal launching pad for my medical career in Britain. One wet August morning, I packed up my bags and set off for the north-east, leaving my wife in Birmingham at her parents' house. The train journey to Newcastle was long, dull and dreary, mainly because it rained all the time, virtually non-stop. I reached the city and took a cab for the hospital to start my work as a registrar. The hospital was a centre for infectious diseases, with a chest and tuberculosis wing, and I was really keen to make a start.

My consultant physician was Dr Karl Verity. He received me and took me round to show me the wards and to introduce me to those already working there. Everyone was courteous, polite and pleasant. I wasn't quite sure if they had ever had an Indian doctor working with them before, but they certainly made this 'New-castle brown' feel at home and I was glad to be in their midst, part of the team. I was living within the confines of the hospital, but could not have the family with me because there was no provision for family accommodation. However, the superintendent of the hospital assured me that arrangements could be made outside the hospital if I chose to have my family over with me.

The following morning, dressed in marshmallow-white clothes, the long doctor's coat on top and stethoscope round my neck, I reported for work and met the sister-in-charge. She took me round the wards and showed me all that there was to be shown to a new doctor. Contrary to expectation, my workload was heavy: treating patients who had been admitted, taking advice from my seniors, giving advice to my juniors, attending to outpatients, doing night work twice a week. It all added up to make my work schedule pretty hectic. But I took it all in my stride because, once again, I was in hospital environs, treating ill patients, trying to make them better.

One morning, as I was crossing the corridors, a woman stopped me and asked if she could see me privately for a few moments to discuss something of a rather personal nature. Being busy at the time, I arranged for her to see me in my office the next day in the afternoon. She arrived spot on time but before she could say anything I warned her that if it was about any of my patients it would have to be with his or her consent.

'No, sir, it's about myself,' she said. 'I want to get married.'

'That's great. Wonderful. But, you see, I'm a registrar of medicine, not marriages,' I told her, wincing with wonderment.

'You see, sir, you don't seem to understand.'

'No, I don't. I really don't.'

'You know Mr X in bed No 16 . . .' she paused, to give me time to connect to the patient.

'Yes,' I said, my mind racing to bed No 16, which was taken up by an elderly man, seriously ill.

'He's my fiancé . . . I want to get married to him. We've been living together for nearly forty years.'

'Living together' was a phrase I wasn't familiar with because it wasn't so common in those days for couples to live together as it is in the dawn years of the twenty-first century. But I decided to figure it out myself or seek someone's help later.

'Mr X would also like to see you tomorrow on this matter. Do you want me to be around at that time?'

'If you want,' I said to her, uncertainly.

As she had predicted, Mr X expressed the desire to see me the next day and I readily consented. He was, after all, a patient of mine. I went to his bed and asked him if he wanted to see me.

'Yes, sir,' he replied, looking at me with his big, melancholic eyes. 'I do.'

'Go right ahead then,' I offered.

'Sir, I've been living with this woman for forty years. I know I'm dying but before I go I'd like to get married.'

'That's fine. Perfectly all right. I'm so pleased for both of you.'

'Sir, you're my doctor. You've been treating me. I want you to be a witness.'

I, a doctor, to be a witness to the marriage of a patient in a hospital ward, my own ward? The request came as a bolt from the blue. No medical book prepares you for situations like that. My books certainly didn't. I thought for a moment and nodded my consent, thinking of him as more than just a patient . . . a human being who had made a request and I had to respond. On human grounds I was one hundred per cent with him but I wasn't quite sure about my position as his doctor. There would also be the legal side, I thought, to be taken into account. I promised to let him know my answer soon.

Later that day I saw the medical superintendent who assured me it was fine if I was to act as a witness in my personal capacity as a doctor but not as a registrar of the hospital.

After the usual formalities had been completed, the marriage ceremony took place in the ward. I found it both pleasant and poignant. Pleasant, because everyone was happy and the ward echoed to the sound of unrestrained, carefree laughter. The bride was all smiles, as brides are on their big day, whether they've been living with their man for forty years or have known him just a few days. It was poignant because the bed-ridden groom was seriously ill, his suffering written on his face. I could tell from his eyes that he was trying hard to conceal his pain. The emotional strain of getting married and the buzz of activity around him had exhausted him and he looked tired.

The ceremony over, the newly-married Mrs X went home alone, to cross the ceremonial threshold herself and not be carried in the arms of her man. We, on our part, sat in our duty room, nibbling bits of the wedding cake, chatting, telling simple jokes, anecdotes and personal experiences about marriages and ceremonies. Funny, isn't it, how on occasions like these, one can always recall someone to whom something outrageously hilarious had happened on their wedding day? My personal feeling about the wedding that I had just been witness to was that Mr X had done the right thing. I had a feeling, sadly, that he had not long to go and had done what in his opinion was the decent thing. A few days later the inevitable happened and he died without ever leaving the hospital bed. The bride of a few days was now a widow, dressed in mourning, trying to come to terms with her grief.

Newcastle at the time was an unhappy city, leagues away from my mental picture of an English town. It was slowly coming out of the trauma of war and dealing, as best as it could, with its aftermath, the physical and psychological scars it had left behind. Scenes of damage and destruction were everywhere – buildings with their guts ripped out, giant craters in the ground, rubble and debris round every corner. Poverty and deprivation stalked the streets. Tuberculosis and chest diseases were rampant and the outpatients' department was clogged with new cases every day. No landscape of hawthorn bushes here; no flowers tumbling out of hanging baskets outside doorways.

I never really settled well there. The hospital wasn't a teaching one and the scope to further one's learning was strictly limited. I got myself a small flat outside the hospital and moved out. My wife and our young daughter joined me and for our Sunday family outings we used to go to Whitley Bay for a seaside stroll, proud parents pushing the baby's pram. We lived there for between six and eight months. In the meantime, I kept looking for another job. I told my consultant about my decision to leave and he said he fully understood my position and even promised to help. The other consultant there was Dr Josef Spitzer, a kind and generous Pole who belonged to the old school of medicine. Soft of speech and modest, he often said that his medical knowledge was confined only to tuberculosis and that he knew nothing about other diseases, though, judging by the few discussions I had with him, nothing could be further from the truth. I admired the quiet way in which he went about his work. During my stay at the hospital, he invited me many times to his house for an evening meal with his family.

In February 1950 I got a letter from the Manchester Regional Health Authority. It was recruiting four trainee senior registrars in chest diseases. Among the scores of job applications I had sent out was one to this authority. It was a huge relief at that time even to be short-listed for an interview as I had built up quite a collection of rejection slips. The interview in Manchester was, by any standard, a daunting affair. Twenty doctors sat bunched together, anxiety levels in orbit, waiting, guessing – 80 per cent of them preordained to go away disappointed, once the outcome was known.

After a few anxious minutes the interview got under way. As usual, we were called in one by one to face the interviewing committee. Not all candidates were asked to wait for the result. Four were asked to stay back and, to my great surprise and delight, I was one of them. Naturally, I was cock-a-hoop to be picked for training as senior registrar for Manchester's chest team.

I went back to Newcastle in a triumphal mood and broke the news to my wife, who was just as pleased over my success. I was now looking forward to the change and she was hopeful of getting a bigger and better home. About two months later, I reported for work at the Manchester Chest Clinic.

Among the doctors starting as trainee senior registrars at the clinic at the same time was Bill Anderson, a jovial Scot with a wry sense of humour. He was already working as a registrar. We became good friends and remained so for a long time. I had to stay in digs for a few days while the family accommodation was being sorted out. My landlady was Mrs Catherine Fox, a no-nonsense woman, hard but fair. Besides breakfast and an evening meal she also took care of my sandwich for lunch, but she made sure I paid for it every day in advance. Now considering I lived there, was a hospital doctor by profession and had virtually all my worldly possessions in the house she owned, I thought this 'no money, no sandwich' rule was a little crusty.

Underneath that rough, tough exterior she harboured a softer, gentler side. My wife, who had temporarily sought refuge with her parents in Birmingham, paid me a visit and Mrs Fox provided her with a room ... of course, with her compliments, and continued to do so on subsequent occasions. Also, so keen was she to see us reunited that she even started to help me in looking for family accommodation. One day she told me she had come to know of a house in Heaton Moor, Stockport, that was available and would suit us fine. I quickly proceeded to meet the land-lord and within minutes I was the tenant of a three-bed furnished semi at the princely sum of £16 a month. Within days we moved in.

At my outpatients' clinic one morning, a young woman came for treatment for tuberculosis. At the time, there were several ways to treat the disease, by antibiotics, artificial pneumothorax and pneumoperitonium. For some unknown reason the clinic had no screening facilities and judging the size of the peritoneum by guesswork was, to say the least, an extremely unsatisfactory and difficult undertaking.

She was sent to have an X-ray and when I looked at the result I was horrified. Not only was she a bad case of tuberculosis, but to make matters more complicated, she was also pregnant, though in the early stages. Feeling sorry and concerned for her, I looked at her, glanced at the X-ray a second time, wishing in my heart what I had just seen wasn't true, and then looked at her again. She could not support the baby while she was being treated for tuberculosis: that was my conclusion. Requesting her to wait for a few minutes, I charged across the road to St Mary's Hospital, a large centre for obstetrics and gynaecology, to seek expert advice. As Professor Richard Morris was busy with his ward round, I had to wait for him in the duty room.

After a few minutes he walked in, tall, dark, handsome, with a cluster of junior doctors in tow. Explaining the position to him, I handed over the envelope containing the X-ray result. He studied the X-ray carefully, engagingly, shook his head and said she couldn't continue with her pregnancy because of her TB. Then, turning to his entourage, he asked one of the juniors to arrange for the next day so that she could be admitted for a 'termination'. I was relieved, for this is what I, too, had thought she needed. Armed with the expert opinion, I dashed straight back to my clinic and the waiting patient.

'Mrs X,' I said to her and went on to explain the problem. 'But you needn't worry. I think we know the solution.' Then I proceeded to map out the details of what we intended to do. She listened with rapt attention, without interrupting.

'So, please come back tomorrow morning, my dear, without taking your breakfast and we'll have you admitted to St Mary's Hospital to terminate the pregnancy. Your treatment will continue after that.'

I expected her to get up, thank me for what I was doing for her and walk out, with a promise to return the following day. But what actually happened took me completely by surprise.

'Can I say something, doctor?' she asked, without moving from her seat.

'Sure, go right ahead.'

'I'm not having the termination,' she said coolly, shaking her head ever so slightly.

I was struck dumb. At a time when young, healthy women were falling over backwards to have a legalised termination, here was one in mortal danger of her life spurning it out of hand – in defiance of my advice, an eminent professor's judgment, and her medical needs.

'If I don't have the termination, will you not treat me?' she asked in a voice barely audible.

I looked at her with some bewilderment and in the ensuing moments recalled the 'comfort for all' part of my medical oath. 'I'm your doctor, young lady. I can't tell you I won't treat you. But the risks in continuing with your pregnancy are enormous, including, possibly, death.' I was blunt. I felt I had to spell it out to her, for it might induce second thoughts.

'I'll take that risk,' she went on, resolutely. 'But you're my doctor and you'll continue to treat me, won't you?'

I nodded. I had given her my opinion and she had chosen to ignore it. Although it hurt, I had to respect her decision. I decided to modify her treatment and monitor the progress, reviewing it every two weeks. While this was going on, I received a call to go to the United States for a year and lost track of her case and, in time, forgot all about it.

Now fast-forward the clock twenty years. I am a consultant physician at Wythenshawe Hospital in Manchester, in charge of the asthma clinic. A woman patient, around fifty, breathing with difficulty, walks into my room and eases herself into the seat opposite me. I examine her, making mental notes and, from time to time, also in writing.

'Do you remember me, doctor?' she asks quite unexpectedly after a while.

I scan her face cursorily, trying to pick up something from my memory bin. Nothing comes back; no bells ring. So I'm forced to tell her, 'I'm afraid . . . it's . . .'

'I was your patient in the chest clinic, oh, a long time ago. You treated me there.'

My mind flashes back to the days at the chest clinic. Still no success. I shake my head slowly, disappointed by the failure of my recall. Before I can speak, she gets up, excuses herself and ambles out of the room. Within no time she's back with a young, handsome, strapping lad by her side.

'See this boy, doctor,' she points to him.

'Yes, a friendly, good-looking fellow,' I reply.

'This is the baby I was expecting when you told me to have a termination.'

Everything races back at the speed of lightning. I know who she is. I'm pleased she's cured of her tuberculosis. I'm also delighted that she did what she did, challenging the odds, defying the enormous risks to herself. I'm glad she ignored my advice. I'm happy she emerged victorious from her ordeal. She's a winner. I doff my hat to her, mentally. What pride! What faith! What love!

Life at the chest clinic was busy. There was a lot of suffering among the people in the city, although materially things were taking a turn for the better. By this time I had also acquired my first car and was using it regularly to go to work. I would leave the vehicle in Denmark Road and go on foot to the clinic from there. One morning, I parked the car, slammed the car door shut with a flourish and then, to my horror, realised that I had left the ignition key inside. Later, I telephoned my wife from the clinic to ask her to bring the duplicate key in the evening. As is her sweet nature, she obliged and turned up at the clinic near the end of the day. Looking a trifle flustered, she went up to my colleague Bill Anderson – I was busy with one thing or another – and explained her quandary to him.

'I was standing next to the car,' she poured out to him, 'when a woman walked up to me and told me to push off as it was her patch. What did she mean by that, Bill?'

Bill presumably had a quiet chuckle to himself and told her it was nothing to worry over and that he would explain later. Then it was my turn. I had to spell it out to her that the street was used regularly by prostitutes for picking up clients. 'She obviously mistook you as a fellow-professional, trying to steal her business. So she told you to move off her patch . . . her territory.'

'The cheek of the woman!' my wife boomed.

'Let's go to my patch, darling,' I said to her with a wicked wink, putting an arm round her waist.

There was no evening work at the clinic and this meant there was plenty of time for going to the cinema, eating out and social soirées. On one of the jaunts I chanced to meet an Indian who had been in Manchester a long time. Sardar Bahadur, a lawyer by profession, had come to Britain in the early 1930s and, like many Indians at the time, wanted to further his education. But somehow he got deflected from his purpose and decided instead to start an Indian restaurant in Manchester – the city's first. His brother, Dar Bahadur, was already a successful restaurateur and was running two eateries in London and Cambridge, thought to be among the first Indian restaurants in the country. So Sardar Bahadur decided to follow his brother's footsteps by opening the Kohinoor in Oxford Street, Manchester.

Sardar was an interesting and enterprising sort of fellow and bonds of friendship soon developed between us. Two or three times a week we would meet at his restaurant for a chat and some 'staff curry' – a light, Indian meal – in his room at the Kohinoor. The conversation usually revolved round the forming of an Indian group with the twin purpose of socialising and promoting Indian culture and way of life, bringing a little bit of India to those Mancunians who could not make it to the sub-continent during the halcyon days of the Raj.

There was already such a body in existence in Manchester but it was moribund and needed kick-starting into life. Sardar had a friend, Dr Homi Anand, a general practitioner, and we all got together along with some other friends and paid half-a-crown each into the kitty – 12p in new money – and so, nearly half a century ago, the first seeds were sown for what is now known as the Indian Association of Manchester, one of the oldest Indian community groups in the country. It has been very active since and, needless to say, moved on to much bigger and better things. My ties with the Indian Association go back to its inception. It is an undiluted love relationship which I have enjoyed and cherished for fifty years. The growth of the association was helped along by Indians who were coming in increasing numbers to work and live in the city in the late fifties and sixties and the Uganda Asians in the seventies.

The presence of an Indian doctor, working virtually in the heart of the city, must have generated some interest among members of the Indian community. On and off they came to see me about their health problems until I discovered that the number of my non-paying private patients was rising faster than I could cope with. Many of them were Sikhs, the hardy, turbaned Punjabis who didn't speak a word of my language, knew only pidgin Hindi and no English at all. They looked to me for succour in matters of health and safety and I, willy-nilly, became their honorary physician. To perform that role with any degree of competence I had to learn a smattering of their language. It was a labour of love but, like all labours of love, it soon began to stretch the demands on my time.

Part of my Sunday routine was to go to their *gurudwara* – temple – for prayer and also to partake in the food following that. By this time we had provided Camille with a little sister, Petula, and the two of them often accompanied me, Camille walking silently on one side and Petula on the other, merrily singing:

> Me and my teddy bear
> Have no worry, have no care
> Me and my teddy bear
> Just play and play all day

While life was proceeding at its merry pace, I received a communication from the American Embassy in London. Apparently, at the time when I was applying for jobs here, there and everywhere, I had sent an application for work in the States. The purpose of the letter was to inform me that I was being considered for a Fulbright Travelling Fellowship to study for a year at a teaching hospital in America and would I attend an interview? I was delighted to hear this. I made my way to London and three days later received a letter to inform me I had been selected to study chest diseases at the Albany Medical College in New York State. My wife was as pleased as I was. By now she was expecting our third child but it was thought to be no hindrance and we agreed that all four of us would go. As the departure date was still some way off, the two of us launched a savings drive of the strictest order. The fellowship would pay for my travel and the family's upkeep in the States, but we still had to find the means to get there and back and enjoy the new country.

CHAPTER 7

An American fellowship

THE EXCITEMENT OF GOING to the United States permeated the whole household. I was keen to find out at first hand how the Americans dealt with their medical problems, especially those in my speciality, while my wife wanted to see the country and experience the American way of life. The nippers, Camille and Petula, were all excited because going to America meant a whole new world opening into their small world. Both of them were often heard talking in conspiratorial tones about which of their favourite toys to take with them. Although the trip was some way off, they considered it a great family venture and played an active role whenever the subject came up for discussion.

My time in Manchester was divided between the chest clinic and home. Although the two of them had their mother's full and undivided attention, I made it a point to spend some time with the children every evening. On my day off, outings were more or less a routine. On Sundays, for example, we would make our way to Belle Vue Zoo to see some of the world's most amazing mammals, reptiles, birds and marine life. The feeding time for the sealions and dolphins and other fish always provided wholesome family entertainment. The girls, one by my side and the other perched on my shoulder, would watch with wide-open, wonder-struck eyes tigers, elephants, giraffes, jaguars and other animals of the wild prowling in their enclosures.

Although life was proceeding at a steady pace, financial worries were always within sight. We were a one-income family, struggling to establish an economic base. We also wanted to buy a home but the housing situation in the city at the time was pretty bad. We were living in rented accommodation, which was just about adequate for us. But the need to move out of the place was forced on us when the landlord let it be known that he was planning to sell the property and we would have to vacate it. My immediate reaction on hearing the news was to buy the place and become owner-occupiers. But there was a big snag – I didn't have the money. My bank balance was pretty anaemic compared to the amount needed to buy the house. Never mind buying outright, I didn't even have enough to put down as a deposit towards the purchase. The landlord was keen to sell the property to me, I was eager to take it off his hands but there lay between us the yawning chasm of money. The sum needed for the deposit was £500. I had no collateral to offer my bank against it and the bank had no intention of advancing the money without it. Result: plenty of anxious moments, head scratching and pacing up and down the lounge.

But in this equation I had somehow forgotten to include one thing: the unexpected. Life has always – well, most of the times, at any rate – been kind to me. It has had a few tricks up its sleeve which it has conjured up from time to time to amaze me and to keep my faith in it. One such occasion was when I had a brief, casual conversation over the garden fence with my neighbour, Thomas Lemere. After the usual preamble about the vagaries of Manchester weather, I chanced to mention my predicament about buying the house and the bank's refusal to advance a loan. As if by magic, those few, by-the-way sentences turned him into an instant heaven-sent genie. He had plenty of assets, such as shares, cash, bonds and things of that financial nature. He did some quick mental calculations and offered to act as my guarantor. He would work out some sort of deal that would meet the bank's requirements and swing the deposit for me. And so, with a few signatures on dotted lines here and there, I was pronounced the owner of the deposit – and therefore the house.

Like Newcastle, Manchester in the early fifties was a wounded and scarred city, emerging from the nightmare of the war. Bomb sites, broken-down buildings and other sorry reminders of the conflict shocked the eyes. There was also overcrowding, and the population suffered from all manner of afflictions. Among them were tuberculosis, asthma and a range of chest diseases. Teams of doctors from the chest clinic used to tour mills and factories regularly, X-raying workers for mass miniature radiography. The programme, I think, lasted nearly two years. I was one of the doctors.

The niggling worry of my impending trip to America was never far away from my mind. I wrote to the Albany hospital a number of times and also had discussions on the telephone with the medical director, Professor John Ericson, about joining him as a junior lecturer in July 1953. Professor Ericson was an American of Swedish descent and was a very helpful person. He advised me on how to prepare for the visit and what to read and also guided me on other, more mundane, non-medical matters. But the most important suggestion that he made was that I should come to America alone first, see for myself how things were, arrange suitable accommodation for the family and then ask my wife and the children to join me.

We had a number of family conferences on the subject. My wife was against it because it meant she would be left alone, an experience she had never previously gone through. If we were in India this problem would not have arisen because of the extended family system which, with its problems in other areas, is a great boon at times like these. There's always somebody to lend a helping hand, share your emotional burden, keep you company. In Britain, although I had my in-laws, and I have no doubt they'd have offered to help us out though it would have been only limited, my father-in-law was getting on a bit. He was also not keeping well. So imposing on them in any way was out of the question.

However, once again, help came from a totally unexpected source. Mary Russell, a nurse at St Mary's Hospital, who was a good friend of my wife and therefore of the family, offered to 'baby sit' for the family until I had made arrangements for them to join me at Albany. Mary, a kind, generous and helpful soul, agreed to come and live in our house, so we finally reached the decision that I would proceed to the United States in June 1953 to take up my fellowship.

Round about the same time, I had problems on the domestic front in India. My father's diabetes was playing up and he was doing virtually nothing about it. At the best of times, he was a difficult patient who spurned medical advice and chose to neglect himself. Even those who were specialists in the field and whom he held in high regard were not exempt from this sort of response from him. For an agonising few days I thought of going to India to see him, even at the risk of putting the American trip in jeopardy. But I was then forced to conclude that it would be a futile exercise because he was in no way going to heed any medical advice from me. For him I'd still be his little son who should know his place in the family and do what he was told.

My passage to America was booked on the *Queen Mary*, a large, luxury Cunard liner. I had to go to London and from there to Southampton to take the ship. I still vividly remember the morning I took the train from Manchester. It was such a wrench. My wife was worried, the girls were tearful and I was just one big emotional knot. Camille kept asking repeatedly if the bungalow I was going to was all right and I repeatedly reassured her that, if the bungalow was all right, I would call the family immediately. But the younger one, Petula, was difficult to control. She cried all morning and as I left home she shouted and screamed that she wanted to go with me. She cared not a jot if the bungalow she had in her mind was okay or not.

On my way to Southampton I met another doctor, Leslie Capel, who, like me, was headed for the United States on the same fellowship but in a different hospital. We got to the port city and I was all set for my first sea journey since arriving in Britain from India nearly six years before. The trip was different, the boat was different, the circumstances were different. I was now an established doctor, working in a hospital, was a family man, had won an American fellowship and felt far more sure of myself. The only gnawing thing was what lay ahead for the next twelve months in a country I had never set foot in before.

The smooth, relaxed atmosphere of the luxury liner made the Atlantic crossing a very pleasant experience indeed. Everything went off swimmingly well and one bright, sunny morning we reached New York. I had to take a train to Albany from there but before that I decided to check out some of the sights and sounds and smells of America's premier city in the few hours I had at my disposal. New York taxi drivers are known for their versatility in catering to the varied demands of millions of tourists who flock to their city or just pass through every year. I've no doubt they make a fine job of it. But if, fifty years ago, there was one rotten apple in the Big Apple in the garb of a cabbie, he was at the steering wheel of my big, yellow taxi. An enormous, burly fellow with a temper as sour as his vinegary face and a penchant for fleecing innocent day-trippers, the unfriendly fellow offered to show me New York for $35. Although the sum was by no means small by those days' standards, I saw the chance as reasonably tempting and threw myself on the back seat with my baggage. Wide-eyed and hungry for the city's landmarks, I kept peering out of the window with curiosity. Barely had we gone round a few blocks when the taxi suddenly shuddered to a halt. My driver and guide informed me that was it. He had shown me all there was to see and he was now ready to take me to Grand Central Station from where I could catch my train. Surprise, surprise, the station was just round the corner.

When he dropped me off, I paid him the money I had agreed with him and – grudgingly – the obligatory gratuity. He counted the five-dollar bills of the tip and fired a verbal volley at me: 'Is that all you can afford?'

'No, but that's all you deserve,' I barked back at him. 'First deserve then desire.' With that openly hostile exchange my brief encounter with New York came to an end and, gingerly, I began to drag my suitcase towards the railway platform.

At Albany station, I looked around half-heartedly but, as I had expected, there was no one with a placard bearing my name, so I made my own way to the hospital where I was received warmly by the sister-in-charge. She told me about arrangements for my stay in an apartment in the hospital compound. Next morning, finally, I came face to face with the man who had been guiding me on matters concerning my work and stay during the period of the fellowship, Professor Ericson. I had had long discussions with him many times in trans-Atlantic telephone calls and had also corresponded with him in some detail. Now I could put a face to the pleasant voice. He was tall, handsome, well-spoken, the sort of person who inspires confidence and would go out of his way to be helpful.

It was a well-run hospital, efficient, business-like, matter-of-fact, and I slotted into it with comfortable ease. I was to act as a resident medical officer for the chest side. Combined with that

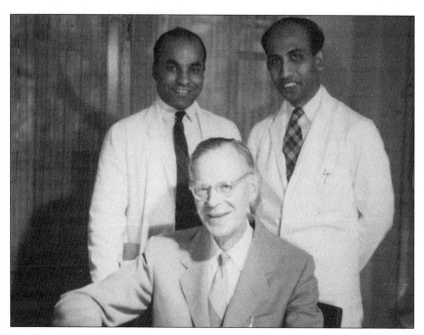

The author (left) in America with Dr Lingapa and (front) Dr Ericson

was my research work and I also had to take care of around 100 in-patients. With the help of two interns, I managed well. One of the interns was Dr David Pender, a promising young man who had just qualified as a doctor. We made a good team. One of the patients in my ward was a young man. One day a letter was handed to him, which contained the bill for his medication. He glanced at it and, making a face, put it under the pillow. When I asked about it, he just shrugged his shoulders and, without revealing the amount, said it would be taken care of. He would hand over the deeds of his house to make the payment. I was amazed by the demand that was being made while he was still receiving treatment and also by his response to it. Under the American system at the time, a patient paid for his treatment in advance while still in the process of getting it.

This was something totally different from the system I had been weaned on, both in India and Britain. However, he wasn't the least perturbed by it because, he said, once he was well and able to resume work, he'd make that kind of money in a matter of a few months. Six to eight, was his estimate, maybe a bit longer. I admired his spirit. You fall over, pick yourself up, flick the dust off your clothes and start walking again. Nothing could be simpler! But I really felt sorry for him, because he was a terminal case.

America was different from what I had seen and experienced in India and in Britain. The Indians become friends easily and, once friendly, they're friends for life. The British are reserved – stiff upper lip and all that. They speak only when spoken to but once they become friends they, too, are friends for forever. Americans, I found, become friends almost at the drop of a hat. Love at first sight, as it were. But bonds of friendship begin to fray at the edges the moment distance puts itself in between. Out of sight, out of mind, as it were. A mild dose of it, certainly.

At work, I had the support of my medical director, co-operation of my colleagues and help of everyone, but outside the hospital boundaries I had no friend to speak of and was missing my wife and the children sorely. I telephoned home at regular intervals but a long-distance chat is a poor substitute for a face-to-face, easy, familiar talk. I wanted them to join me and asked my wife to get the money out of the bank and book the passage. In October 1953, they set sail from Southampton for New York. I travelled by train from Albany to meet and greet the four of them – by this time there had been a welcome addition to the family in the form of a son – at the pier.

My wife was really courageous, for it takes a brave woman to undertake the boat trip with two lively girls and a babe-in-arms. All that preparation, all that planning, all that work. Her 'to do' list must have looked like a plan to invade a small country. But she did it and did it admirably. When the four of them arrived in America, I had already moved to a bungalow outside the hospital. The girls joined the local school and life gradually got back on an even keel, though the backdrop was different. It was a pretty enjoyable time once again.

I worked hard and we travelled at every opportunity that came our way. We made a crop of good friends along the way. The girls captivated the Americans with their cute English accent. Some of them made the two say certain words over and over again because they liked the way they said them. Time flew at a fast and furious pace and the stage arrived when we had to start thinking of returning to England. During my stay at Albany, I had learned a lot and I also had had a small operation on my spine which, I felt, was a bit of a setback to an otherwise faultless 'year out.'

It was a happy homecoming when we got back to Manchester. I was looking forward to sliding back into the old routine, as I still had my contract with the chest clinic. We got off the train that had brought us from London. A light drizzle was falling when we came out of the railway station and we did not have a single umbrella between us but, for once, it did not matter. We were back home at last and we had brought with us pleasant and happy memories by the bagful.

CHAPTER 8

Baguley and Wythenshawe Hospitals

A COUPLE OF DAYS after returning from the United States, I reported for work to Baguley Hospital, Manchester, instead of to the chest clinic, as I had been reassigned there. The change was necessitated by reorganisation that had taken place while I was away. I knocked gently on the door of the hospital superintendent and got a pleasant surprise. Extending his hand in my direction was none other than Dr Tom Wilson. He was lording it over a large table, the master of all he surveyed in the big room. His face lit up with a huge smile.

'Welcome back, Dr Chatterjee,' he said, with his usual Scottish affability.

'It's great to be back, indeed,' I answered, as we shook hands.

'And how was the States?'

'It was united when I got there and it was still united when I left,' I said in a dead-pan sort of way.

'How droll.' He gave a raucous guffaw.

'I spent twelve months there, Tom, I can't sum it up in twelve words.'

'Fine. First instalment at lunchtime, then.'

Dr Wilson was the new superintendent of the hospital. It was a recent appointment and, in my judgment, they couldn't have picked a better person for the job. He was forward-looking, fair and open-minded. We talked briefly about ourselves, our families and then, the pleasantries out of the way, the subject turned to the hospital. He fixed his gaze on me and told me that I had been posted under him as a senior registrar.

'I'm grateful for the opportunity,' I replied. 'You know I'll do my best for the hospital and the patients.'

'I know you will. I know you well. I'm looking forward to a long and happy association with you.'

The new hospital was large, scattered and, in my opinion, a little unwieldy. The reason for this was that in its previous incarnation it was a sanatorium and had been converted into a hospital in phases over a period of time, not necessarily with the best results in certain areas. During one of my many job interviews, I had been told that Baguley was a hospital to watch as it was heading for the heights and would some day be one of the biggest hospitals in the city. Decades later when I left it, the prophecy had indeed come true. I consider myself fortunate that I was able to contribute in a small way towards its development. The day-to-day pressures at the hospital were within manageable levels. I had an outpatients' clinic and also had to look after two wards, mainly for tuberculosis patients, with a smattering of those suffering from other chest diseases. A junior doctor was there to assist me and we made an excellent team. Once a week we had a ward round, with the superintendent as head of the pack. It was mainly a stiff, formal exercise.

At work one day, I received a telephone call from Dr Robert Arland, who was a general practitioner in Stockport, not very far from where I lived. He had heard about me and wanted to know if I would assist him in his surgery on a part-time basis. I could not, obviously, commit myself there and then on the phone, so I told him that I would give him my decision in a day or two. I had a word with the hospital superintendent and he assured me it was fine as long as the extra work did not interfere with my official duties at the hospital. After a brief consultation with my wife at home, I made up my mind that I'd accept the position.

Dr Arland's surgery was in an old house which had been converted into a practice. The doctor himself was a pleasant bachelor, who took good care of his patients. My life was now run along strict lines. The day was taken up by work at Baguley Hospital. I would then come home for tea and spend some time with the family and then proceed for my evening surgery at the end of which I would return home with £5 in my back pocket – a good amount by those days' standards.

Coming home from Stockport one night, I chanced to spot a young lad, of Indian appearance, walking towards the town hall disconsolately, looking forlorn and lost. I stopped the car and asked if everything was all right with him. He gave a non-committal shrug as if he didn't know what to say. It was accompanied by a wry smile and he introduced himself.

'I'm Gopala Krishnan,' he offered.

'You mean Gopal?' I asked.

'I'm a South African citizen, of Indian origin,' he went on. 'Therefore it's Gopala.' And he explained who he was and what had brought him to that part of the north of England. He had finished his schooling in Stockport but was encountering enormous problems in his attempt to pursue his education at university level because he came from a poor family in Durban and the South African government was unwilling to sponsor him for higher education because of its policy on race.

I felt the young man needed a break from his problems and asked him if he would like to come to our house, meet my family and have something to eat. He was more than willing and eased himself into the passenger seat. By the time we got home, it was nearly 10 o'clock. I asked my wife if she could rustle up some food for the visitor. A line cut into her forehead as she exclaimed, 'Food, at this hour!' A pause. Then the line disappeared as quickly as it had appeared. 'Food, of course. Would you like some fish curry and rice?' she asked turning to Gopala. It wasn't the first time I had inflicted unexpected guests on her, though seldom so late in the day. About half an hour later, as he tucked into a pile of steamed rice and hot fish curry, Gopala reeled out his life story. His forefathers had migrated to South Africa years before. His father, who had a humble grocery shop in Durban, had died at a young age and his mother, who had ambitions of giving her children the best possible education they could get, was forced to take up the reins of the business.

Indians at the time were not looked upon favourably in South Africa and the government had slapped all sorts of checks and controls on them. As the restrictions meant that they were even denied access to good education, so Gopala's mother had decided to send him to England for studies. He had successfully completed his school and was ready to go to university. Unfortunately, the family lacked the means to support him and the government lacked the will to sponsor him because he was the wrong colour. I was appalled and filled with ire at the discriminatory official position his government had adopted and felt sorry for the victim of it, who sat so innocently at my dining table, eating fish curry and rice and pouring out his heart to us. Apart from sympathy and food that evening, I also promised to help him in any way I could. Little did I know at that time how difficult it would be to help someone whose own government had so callously abandoned him to his fate.

I knew a number of people in a position of influence at the university and other places and decided to have a word with them. Among them was Sir Robert Platt, professor of medicine, one of the kindest people I've had the good fortune to meet in my life. I told Sir Robert about the young South African who wanted to study medicine but had neither the independent means nor his country's support for doing so. Weeks passed without any positive response from any quarter and I was beginning to feel a bit dejected when one evening the telephone rang at home. At the other end was Sir Robert, who wanted to know if the young man was still available as, if so, he had something in mind for the South African. I informed Gopala who proceeded more or less immediately to meet Sir Robert at Manchester Royal Infirmary. Three days later he started work as a technical assistant in the professor's research team. This was an act of great generosity on the professor's part and I will never forget it. It opened a window of opportunity for a deserving young man who hadn't had much luck in life before.

Our house was gradually becoming a centre for Manchester's Indian student community. Regularly, they appeared on the doorstep, needing help of one kind or another. Some turned up just for a chat and a cha. As we were never short of these young visitors, my wife was never short of baby-sitters.

Apart from the students, my involvement with the Indian community as a whole was also taking deeper roots. The Indian Association that we had founded a couple of years before was now fully operational, doing admirable work in integration, 'bridge-building' and bringing glimpses of Indian culture to the local population. We now also had the help and assistance of a number of businessmen. We would meet regularly at the Ceylon Tea Centre on Oxford Road, near the city's central library. Among the businessmen lending us their support were Govind Ruia, Mulshanker Oza, Babubhai Kapadia, Brij Kapoor and Jyoti Parkash, all of them affluent, prospering in the rag trade and mindful that they also had a key role to play in the life of the community and the city.

Besides these stalwarts, there were young idealists, university and polytechnic students who included Narendra Gulhati and his English wife Anna. Anna was young, pleasant, and full of bright ideas. We became friends and continue to be so to this day. Gulhati, who worked for War on Want for a while, now successfully runs his own travel agency while Anna is a psychotherapist.

While I was making steady professional progress, I received a telephone call from the hospital superintendent asking me for a chat. During the course of the meeting he revealed that the post of deputy superintendent was shortly to be advertised and he wanted me to apply for it. I was very pleased and terribly excited that he had me in mind for that position. It was not difficult to see why. I had a good medical background, possessed a postgraduate qualification from Britain and plenty of experience. Apart from this, I had spent a year in the United States honing my skills. To be honest, even I did not see any hurdles in my way. So, following Dr Wilson's suggestion, I duly applied for the job of deputy superintendent and, as expected, was short-listed for an interview. On the day of the interview, I spruced myself up and, bristling with confidence, entered the interview room. I took a fleeting look at the interviewing panel. Some of the faces were familiar, the superintendent among them, while others were new to me. After a long and grilling interview, I was told I had been unsuccessful. When I came to know who had been appointed, I was crushed. In my estimation, I was a better candidate − if not by a mile, certainly by a fair distance. But then, he was not an Indian and I was.

I came home and broke the news to my wife. As is her wont, she tried to pep me up, offering words of encouragement. It was not the end of the world, she said. Also, it wasn't the first time that I had been turned down for a job. I had succeeded more times than I had failed and I would succeed again. All this helped to ease my disappointment. Next day at work, I saw the hospital superintendent.

'I'm sorry you didn't get the job,' he sympathised, before I could say anything. 'You were, of course, the best candidate and I'm sure if your name was Smith or Jones or Taylor or Brown, you would've got it.'

I never thought that discrimination like that happened in the medical world, a profession that I had always regarded as being in the upper echelons of society. Discrimination is like sex; it does not happen in high society, does it? I had never heard such a frank admission of race bias from anyone before and coming from someone as close as Dr Wilson, who doubtless had supported my candidature during the interview, didn't make it less painful.

'Don't be disheartened, old chap, and also don't go round looking for another job,' he advised me in a firm voice. 'Stay here. There's bound to be another opening sooner or later. I'd like you to reapply.'

His words acted as a balm and lifted the gloom further. About three months later another opportunity arrived, this time for the post of a physician. I seized it. I applied for it and I got it. I was full of gratitude to the superintendent for his encouragement. My wife, as usual, was more than delighted with my progress. Consultant posts, about fifty years ago, were difficult to come by. A physician's position was a stepping stone to it. I had started as a tuberculosis physician at Baguley and was moving forward. I now had a permanent position and a guaranteed, regular income. The new position also signalled a change in direction to the surgical side and provided me with an opportunity to carry out research in my field. I told the hospital superintendent about my desire to do some research work. This meant setting up a respiratory physiology unit – a sort of laboratory. Not only did he like the idea instantly, he told me that he had been thinking of doing something along those lines for a long time.

'Listen,' he added, with some seriousness, 'why don't you start a respiratory unit while I think of an intensive care unit?'

With great enthusiasm we shook hands on the pact – the fifties' equivalent of the new century's high five – and that marked the beginning of finding ways and means to negotiate the tortuous humps and bumps, twists and turns of red tape in order to get the project off the ground. I found out that there was a firm in London operating under the name of P. K. Morgan and Co that specialised in equipment for respiratory diseases. I got in touch with them and the company chief, Mr Morgan, a pleasant young man, came to see me and said he would do everything possible to help us but he was pretty firm on one thing: any equipment the unit needed would have to be paid for. It was for sale and not to be given away free of any charge.

Naturally, to procure funds, I had to approach the Regional Health Authority. Their initial response was non-committal. However, I detected that some members of the authority showed an interest in the scheme and wanted more details. One member even assured me – strictly in confidence of course – that the project was worth taking up and money would have to be found for it sooner or later. He advised me to persevere with it. He was right. A small sum of money soon materialised and with the active support of the hospital superintendent the unit eventually came to life in a little room by the side of a ward. Today, I'm glad to say, it rubs shoulders with some of the country's top establishments in the field.

As the news about the respiratory physiology unit spread, one of the surgeons working in the hospital, Mr Frank Nicholson, came to see me and told me about a similar but well established laboratory that was doing outstanding work in Malmö, Sweden. He rhapsodised so much about the Swedish operation that I was forced to take the address of the place from him and wrote to its doctor in charge, Dr Lavé Svenberg. I told him about my own modest operation at Baguley and asked him if I could visit the Malmö District General Hospital and spend some time doing research work there.

Promptly, in less than a week, he responded, expressing delight at my idea and offering all kinds of help and assistance. There was just one small hitch: his hospital could not pay for the time I was going to spend in Malmö. However, I would be treated as a guest of the hospital and as such would be entitled to all other facilities, like board and lodging and access to facilities of the laboratory. It seemed a perfectly reasonable arrangement to me. After all, I was going there to do my own work and pick up ideas on how to make my own unit better and more efficient.

I asked the Regional Health Authority for leave of absence for three months. Silence. No answer for a month. Then came a curt reply, telling me I could have three months off with pay but the money would be deducted after I returned from Sweden and resumed my duties. I didn't know what to make of the attitude. Three months' pay to be docked because I was trying to bring improvements in the way our hospital treated its patients! The hospital superintendent was equally baffled but told me to go right ahead with the project. As for the deduction of pay, we would cross that bridge when we came to it.

In early March 1957, I set off for Gothenburg by boat. The winter was bone-chilling. For the first time in my life I saw frozen sea. It was really a curious sight on a cold, clear, freezing morning when our ship approached Gothenburg. An ice-breaker inching in front led us into the harbour. With shivering hands I pushed down a Swedish breakfast of cold fish, spinach and boiled egg, and proceeded by train to Malmö where I was warmly received by Dr Svenberg at the station. He apologised in advance if the hospital accommodation did not measure up to my expectation. He had arranged it because it was in close proximity to the laboratory and therefore I wouldn't have to waste time travelling every morning and evening. However, if I wanted to change it he would do his best to find me another place.

The laboratory was equipped with state-of-the-art technology of the era. The building was spick and span, bright and cheerful, roomy and well laid-out – the sort of place that invites one to spend a lot of time in it. That, precisely, was my motive. The people who worked there were friendly, helpful and eager to assist me in my work. Although I did not know a word of Swedish and their knowledge of English was somewhat limited, we managed quite well. In the process, I made many friends and learned as much physiology as I possibly could.

Most of my weekends were spent with Dr Svenberg, his wife Britt and their two children at their house. Britt was a pleasant and attractive woman with a friendly disposition and she went out of her way to make me feel at home. One Saturday morning, towards the end of my stay in Malmö, she decided to lay on a special treat for me. Britt got a few spices together and announced that she was going to cook a curry dinner. She requested that I should help her in preparing the meal. Nothing intricate. Just which spices to use, when and how much. Things of that nature. So, following her bidding, I rolled up my sleeves and mucked in with my contribution to the chicken curry. By the afternoon, the feast was ready to be laid on the table. Instead, they decided that we would pack the food and head for the family's winter chalet in the forest. We got to the chalet and the food was spread out on the table. Flowers were placed and candles were lit. We said grace and tucked in. The rice was on the lumpy side and I bet they'd never tasted goulash like that before in their life.

CHAPTER 9

Continental travel

W HILE IN SWEDEN I spent a lot of time alone. Part of the
reason for this was the nature of my work. I had gone there
with certain projects and, as the time frame to see them through
was limited, I had to get tightly engrossed in the research. But
partly it was enforced upon me because, when the work was
finally over for the day, everyone in the department had gone
home and there was no one around to socialise with, to have a
friendly chat. But it posed no major problem as I'm not averse to
my own company. I enjoy reading biographical accounts of world
leaders and people who, whatever their field of endeavour, have
made achievement the central core of their life.

The research work I was doing was very rewarding. I had the
full run of the hospital laboratory and the help of an extremely
cooperative staff and learned a lot about the work that was being
done in Sweden in my speciality. Dr Svenberg and his wife Britt
were a charming couple and they made a point of inviting me to
their house to entertain me whenever I needed a break from my
work. In time, I got to know them and their two children very
well.

While there were still a few days left for my work, Britt
suggested that, if possible, I should call my family to join me. She
was keen that we should see a bit of Sweden and also take in part
of the continent. In those days, overseas holidays were still a
privilege of the few and a rarity for working men and women.
Air travel was not as common as it is today and it was also
ferociously expensive. But my work was proceeding nicely and I
had made great progress. I was, therefore, in a fortunate position
to combine leisure with a bit of pleasure for the rest of my stay
in Sweden. The only snag was money. But then money, I
suppose, has always been an obstacle for people in my position,
especially in the early stages of their career when they are
struggling to get somewhere. 'Ah, well, a money problem is

84

something most of us are born with and so if I don't take a chance the opportunity will be lost.' With this thought in mind, I decided to throw caution to the wind and telephoned home to find out what my wife thought of the idea of a holiday on the continent with the family. As expected, she jumped at the chance. It was agreed that she would bring the children and the car to Sweden by boat and we would make Malmö the starting point of our journey.

The children, always great holiday fun, were also out of their cotton socks with joy. Though young in years, they were adventurous, cooperative and adaptable as far as foreign travel was concerned. As a family, we've often had great times together, laughed together and, on the odd occasion, cried together. So, one morning a telegram arrived to tell me that the boat tickets had been booked and the family would be arriving on a certain day. So things were now well and truly on the move and I was really looking forward to the holiday.

During my stay at Malmö, I had made numerous friends, among them Helge Woolf, professor of surgery at the hospital. He asked me to a party he was hosting on 1 August. It is an important day in the Swedish calendar. It marks the start of the holiday season and begins with a feast of crayfish, known as the kräftskiva. It's a truly great occasion. Friends and family gather for a party, a lot of crayfish is cooked and pushed down with enormous amounts of drink, mainly Swedish schnapps. The schnapps are usually very potent and set your mouth and throat on fire as they make their journey inside you, but once they reach their destination, they're a heaven of delight.

The professor's party was a marvellous occasion. The whole of his department was present, as were some members from other units. We all sailed to an island off Malmö where we spent the festive evening. With my limited knowledge of Swedish customs, I thought crayfish was the only item on the menu and, like a fool, helped myself to generous portions of it and the bread and schnapps that accompanied it. As I was nearly full, the main course arrived amid a lot of cheering – succulent, inch-thick steak with mouth-watering trimmings, vegetables and what-have-you. That evening I discovered that ignorance may be bliss on any other subject, but when it comes to food it certainly puts you at a serious disadvantage. The merry-making went on until the early hours by which time there were legless bodies all over the place, asleep in whichever position they collapsed. For me it was truly a memorable experience.

Two days later my family arrived and I met them at the quayside. I had gone there with Mons Arborilious, a junior doctor from our department. In glorious, early-morning sunshine on a cold day we had set off from Malmö to Gothenburg. He had offered to drive me there. The plan was that on the way back I would follow him in order to build up my confidence for driving. The children were bursting with excitement at being in Sweden. By the time we got back to Malmö it was night, but the sun was still shining in all its glory, a strange sight for the eyes to behold. We stayed in Sweden a few days, having an exciting time. Then we bid our fond farewell to that wonderful Scandinavian country and headed in the direction of Denmark.

During that period I received the sad news from India that my father had passed away. Although I had not seen him since I left India in 1947, the loss was still too great. I was utterly devastated. Suddenly, I felt lonely, and bitterly I cried, with no one to share my grief. There was also considerable anger in me – against my brothers who had failed to keep me informed about his deteriorating health. Thousands of miles away from Patna, for me, one minute he was there and the next minute he was gone. It made the shock worse. If nothing else, he was a great psychological prop and that prop had now been taken away from me.

We crossed the sea and arrived in Copenhagen. The city was like the backdrop of some Hans Christian Andersen fairy tale. We all found it, as the song goes, wonderful. While we were there, Dr Svenberg and Britt joined us for a brief vacation and their arrival added to the good time we were all having. From Copenhagen we proceeded to Hamburg and found the city rising from the ashes of the war. A lot of construction was going on everywhere, a lot of rebuilding activity in evidence. Our next stop was Breda, a small Dutch town known for its potteries. From Holland we drove to France and finally we crossed the Channel and arrived back in Britain.

We were thoroughly exhausted but also terribly excited that we had managed to see so many countries in just a single trip. It was early August and I was glad to be going home. I was merrily driving to Manchester when a policeman flagged me down. The reason: I was on the wrong side of the road. When I told him we were returning from a holiday in Europe where people had this nasty habit of driving on the wrong side and bad habits are easily picked up, he smiled and waved me on with a cautionary word. I settled back into the old routine quickly enough. My job at Baguley was proceeding satisfactorily and I had gathered more knowledge in Malmö about respiratory physiology to take my work forward. While in Sweden I had made copious notes and a list of equipment I would need for my work in Manchester. A few days later I gave a report to the Regional Health Authority on the progress I had made and also my 'shopping list' to expand our research laboratory at the hospital. The regional medical officer didn't seem terribly impressed by the report. He promised nothing, merely stated he would do what he could. I came away from the meeting deflated. Dr Wilson, who was also present at the meeting, however, wasn't downhearted. He asked me to persevere with the project because, as he saw it, we were making progress, albeit at a lamentably slow pace. How right he was! Within days I saw clear signs of things turning in our favour.

While I was in Sweden, Dr Wilson had received a letter from the state government of West Bengal who had made me an offer of a senior position in Calcutta Medical College. He had forwarded this information to me and I wrote back to Calcutta to say that I'd like to discuss the matter further, possibly on a visit to India that I was shortly planning to make. This was a period marked by many opportunities I had and many opportunities that I missed. Three offers came from India offering senior positions, while in Britain I had been classified as a physician doing a consultant's work. I was paid extra for the extra responsibilities and had been promised that in the fullness of time I would be made a pukka consultant.

While I was mulling over the Calcutta opening, I received an invitation to give three lectures on respiratory physiology in Bombay. At precisely the same time invitations also arrived from

Delhi, Calcutta and Patna to speak on medical matters. With so many speaking invitations and job offers on the table, it was extremely difficult to resist the temptation of paying the old country a visit. A long period had elapsed since I had left India and so many changes had taken place in my life. So, with India weaving its magic, I applied for and got leave of absence for six weeks. Coming to England from Bombay, I had taken the sea route but, going to Bombay from England, air was my preferred method as I had only limited time at my disposal. I had never flown such a long haul before. The plane made three stops, at Rome, Beirut and Delhi en route to Bombay, picking up petrol and passengers, I guess. And so, on a bright, sunny and warm day, under a spotlessly blue sky, I arrived in India's financial centre to renew my acquaintanceship with Bombay, the city I had left way back in 1947.

A clutch of doctors was present at Santa Cruz airport to welcome me and I felt really important to see so many of them present to meet and greet me. Arrangements for my stay had been made at the Taj, a hotel with a legendary status and ranked at the time as one of the best in the world. It was flattering, indeed, to be accorded such cordial treatment. I was made to feel a VIP all the way. During my stay in Bombay, I met a number of people from the medical world, including top experts like Dr Aaga Singh Kochar and Dr Paul Anand.

From Bombay I flew to Delhi and checked into the hotel that had been booked for me. It was a modest affair compared with the Taj but quite comfortable. The next thing on my personal itinerary was to get in touch with my old-time friend Dr Kamta Bhargava, who was working in the Railway Hospital in New Delhi and lived in Bhagwandas Road, one of the better localities in the city. We agreed to meet at his place for a bite to eat and also to meet his family. We had not seen each other for well over eleven years and I was sure a lot must have happened to him in that time as it had to me. Eleven years, after all, is a sizeable chunk of time in one's life. Armed with a bouquet of roses, I knocked on his door in the evening and was greeted by an ebullient thirty-something who extended a warm, welcoming hand in my direction and introduced herself as Shanta Bhargava, Kamta's wife. A charming and attractive Kashmiri, she was also a medic.

After a brief exchange of pleasantries in the entrance hall, she awarded me the freedom of the house with words to the effect that I was free to stay for as long as I liked and was at liberty to come and go as I pleased. For me, it was like being awarded the freedom of the city. With friendly jollity, she mildly reprimanded me for not coming to the Bhargava household straight from the airport but accepted my explanation that I was a guest of the medical fraternity in Delhi and all arrangements for my stay plus most of my itinerary had been made by my hosts. However, there was always a next time.

The dinner was highly enjoyable. The whole family, including Nalin and Hemant, their two sons, and daughter Neera, sat around the table, occasionally eyeing me with cherubic curiosity. Relaxed atmosphere, congenial company, recollections of the times past punctuated with belly laughs, echoes of a reunion, mouth-watering comestibles – my favourite fish curry among them – what more could I ask for? It was truly a memorable occasion. These family occasions, I find, have a great charm. There's something festive about them. Neera, a pleasant and smart young person, volunteered to take me on a tour of the city and show me some of its historic sights.

The Delhi visit over, I headed for Patna by train. I had not travelled on an Indian train – still chugging along nicely in the steam era – for a long time and I was really looking forward to the experience. Half the time during the journey, I was peering out of the window as a vast landscape of dry and dusty plains, bridges, fields, rivers, whizzed past to the click-a-clack rhythm of the wheels for nearly two days. At Mughal Sarai, not very far from Patna, my brother joined me on the train. He had also brought his two daughters, Stella and Gopa, with him. The young girls were carrying garlands of marigold flowers in their hands to welcome me. I found the gesture moving.

In Patna, we all piled into a taxi and went to my brother's home. I spent the next few days there and the family looked after my every creature comfort. During the stay, I paid a visit to my old Alma Mater and gave a lecture on my speciality, which was received with enthusiasm. It was a great feeling being back on home ground as a 'local boy made good'. Most of the professors and senior lecturers who had taught me were still in their posts. Wherever I went I was received with open arms and plaudits were heaped on me. It was a hectic time and I was swept off my feet by my numerous engagements. No two lunches or dinners were in the same place. Sometimes even the breakfast was taken up by a meeting. There were parties aplenty in my honour and the hospitality shown towards me was truly amazing and, at times, overwhelming. Among the series of meetings I had was one with Dr Bistu Mukerjee and his wife Annie, who was a sister-in-charge during my college days. We sat and chattered the whole time.

Calcutta was the next stop. The same old routine – a series of lectures, meetings, receptions, endless handshakes and what-have-you. But there were one or two notable differences. A meeting had been arranged with the Chief Minister of the state, Dr B. C. Roy, and with Colonel B. Chakraborty, director general of medical services, West Bengal. The encounter with Dr Roy was a daunting one. I had never before in my life met anyone of that high calibre and standing in the political world. Apart from being the Chief Minister, he was also a well-known doctor and an ardent Congress Party worker. It was arranged that I should see him in his office. Silently, I was ushered into his room where, at the end of a large table, sat the Bengali leader, an imposing figure.

He welcomed me and after the usual preliminaries asked, 'Tell me, when are you going to join us?'

'I will, sir,' I replied. 'I have to complete my tour first.'

'You come and join us and we'll help you all the way.'

I nodded, unable to give any firm commitment.

'A letter will be sent to you in a day or two at your England address. When you get back there you'll see it. It's an invitation for you to join Calcutta Medical College as a professor.'

'I'm grateful to you for thinking so highly of me. I shall certainly give it serious thought.'

He also promised that I was free to acquire any equipment that I needed for the department, irrespective of the cost. Such carte blanche made the offer seem very attractive and I was tempted to give an affirming nod. I asked if it would be possible for me to have study leave for a few days before deciding. Even this request was met with a swift and positive response.

I came back to Britain happy with my accomplishments and wondering quite seriously whether to take up the professorship in Calcutta. A prestigious job in Bengal's prestigious medical college was something for which any Bengali doctor would have given his right hand. It was the stuff dreams are made of. For me, however, the offer had a downside too. My children had moved from nursery to primary schools. They were doing well and were keen to continue in the same environment. In any future plans that I made for myself, I had now to consider their education too. I knew what a pivotal role education had played in my life and I was keen that they should have every opportunity to pursue their own. At least they should acquire some qualification or skill which would stand them in good stead should, God forbid, they hit bad times.

Besides this, I now had my own department and a research team. I had been given the position of a consultant physician, one of just a handful of doctors from the Indian sub-continent who enjoyed that privilege. It was important, too, that I should take the research work I had started at Baguley further. I also had a

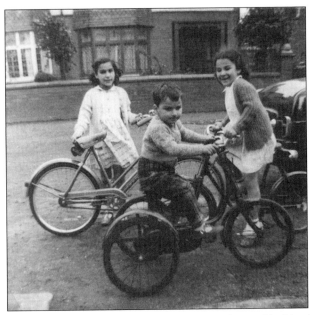

Camille (left), Petula and Nigel in Heaton Moor, Stockport, Cheshire, in 1958

large private practice, including many non-paying patients. My involvement with the Indian community in Manchester was quite deep. So, taking all these factors into account, agonisingly painful though it was, I decided to decline the professorship in Calcutta.

CHAPTER 10

Gandhi Hall

L IFE IN MANCHESTER had moved up a gear. I was now a fully-fledged consultant physician and as such my hospital workload was increasing. I had my private practice, too. Proceeding side by side with these commitments was my research work. Also, I was gradually spreading my wings in the treatment of diseases that were outside my speciality. At the same time, a number of pharmaceutical companies had approached me to try out new drugs they were working on and that had its own attraction. All this meant a hectic daily work schedule. My day started early and, on most days, I didn't get home until late. But being in the thick of things also brought new challenges and satisfaction when these challenges were successfully met.

Socially, too, the pace was busier. The Indian Association had no fixed abode of its own and members met wherever they could find a venue. At the time, there was only one Indian restaurant in Manchester, the Kohinoor, on Oxford Road. Its proprietor, Mr Sardar Bahadur, was good enough to open his doors to the association, which held its meetings there. By this time, students from India were arriving in increasing numbers to study in the city's universities, mainly UMIST. They also actively participated in these meetings, which included important dates in the Indian calendar, such as the Republic Day, Independence Day and major Hindu festivals, like *Holi* and *Diwali*. These main events were usually celebrated at the Midland Hotel as it could accommodate a lot more people. Members also gathered in a number of homes, where musical concerts by visiting artists were held and home-cooked Indian food was served. Chicken tikka masala, far from being the national dish, wasn't even on the back burner at the time and the spicy home-made fare often proved to be the highlight, especially with the student community. These regular get-togethers went some way towards alleviating their loneliness and helped them cope better with the pressures of education in a new country.

During one such meeting at a friend's house, I suggested to the few members present that, in view of the growing number of Indians in Manchester and the interest being shown in the work of the association, it was important that it should end its nomadic existence and find a place of its own. This would be its base where members could meet on a regular basis. A permanent address and telephone number were also prerequisites if the association was to expand its activities. Heads nodded in approval, glances were exchanged and whispers were hissed. It was obvious the idea had its appeal – the question was who would take up the torch. I proposed that we should raise money towards the purchase of a house. To set the ball rolling I put my hand in my pocket and got my wallet out. Such was the enthusiasm for the project that within no time we had collected enough to put down a deposit towards the purchase of a property.

As luck would have it, a couple of days later a friend, Harold Wolestencroft, who was a financial adviser, telephoned me about something else. During our conversation he mentioned that there was a hall up for sale and in his opinion it was definitely worth a look. We agreed to meet and went to see the place in Brunswick Road, Withington. It belonged to the Latter Day Saints who used it for holding their meetings. They wanted £16,000 for it – way over the association's budget. Mr Wolestencroft suggested that we negotiate the price and, in order to show that we were serious about buying it, have the property surveyed.

A surveyor was commissioned and he had a good look at the hall. In his report he suggested that the hall's realistic price was around £9,000. Armed with the recommendation, Mr Wolesten-croft approached the owners on the association's behalf and offered £10,000 for it. To our great surprise the offer was accepted and we decided to buy the place outright. A drive to raise funds started in top gear and quickly went into overdrive. Beg, borrow or steal tactics were adopted. We organised a raffle, with tempting prizes like two return tickets to the old country by courtesy of Air India – the business community chipped in handsomely – morning coffees, late-night dinners. You name it, we did it. Within a matter of days, the meeting place of the Latter Day Saints became Gandhi Hall. It was decided that in future all important Indian functions would be held there. Gandhi Hall was officially opened in March 1969 by the High Commissioner for India and in attendance were local Lord Mayors and MPs and many other dignitaries and political figures.

Enlarged, improved, refurbished, it's fully operational to this day. It's a matter of great pride to me that I belong to the founding group who took the Indian Association forward in the early stages of its formation. The association is vitally important to me. I am proud of being a part of Manchester's Indian community and the community, in turn, has given me enough love, affection and respect to last a lifetime. Later on, Labour came into power and local MPs such as the late Sir Leslie Lever and Lord Orme became keenly interested in the work of the association and gave their whole-hearted support to it. The hall today is home to the Radha Krishna Temple and a focal point of Hindu religious activities. The temple even has its own resident priest who performs all the rites and ceremonies and the Sunday service in particular is well attended. Other users in the past have been Manchester's Indian senior citizens who, after many years, have moved out to more suitable premises for their growing needs. Its latest users are the Bengali Cultural Society who celebrate *Durga* and *Kali puja* and events allied to religious events in the Bengali calendar. It is also let out for some private social functions and marriage ceremonies.

While the augmentation of the Indian Association was pro-ceeding smoothly, the number of Indian students in my 'supervi-sion' was also increasing. One such student was Ram Gopal Mehra, who had come to study textile technology at UMIST. He would routinely come to our house every Saturday and spend some time with us. This arrangement continued for a while until one weekend he failed to turn up. Dismissing it as just a minor aberration, we thought nothing of it. Come the next weekend and Ram Gopal was again conspicuous by his absence. We telephoned him at his 'digs' in Didsbury but there was no response. Concerned, I decided to pay him a visit one evening after finishing my work at the hospital. When I managed to reach him, he was lying face down in his bed with what he described as a 'severe headache.' The lights in his room had not been turned out and the impression I got was it had been like this for some time. I immediately decided to take him to hospital. He was admitted straightaway and a consultant colleague of mine came to see him and later telephoned me at home to say the patient was seriously ill with tubercular meningitis. His treatment would begin after the results of the tests carried out on him were available.

It's a serious disease and I was really worried, so I telephoned his parents in Bombay and suggested that, as he was married, his wife come over forthwith to look after him. He needed full-time attention. Within days his wife, Snehlata, arrived and began a bedside vigil on her husband which lasted weeks. With proper medication and her devoted care, Ram Gopal was soon on the mend. It took some six months before he was fit again and able to resume his studies. As a consequence of the serious nature of his illness and the time he had been away from the college, he had to settle for an M.Sc. degree instead of the Ph.D. which was his original aim. But we were all mightily relieved that he was well and had accomplished at least part of his mission.

While my involvement with the Indian community was increasing, the Indian Association elected me as its president and I remained in that position for a considerable period of time. My participation in local politics also saw a big upward curve. The Labour movement was gathering momentum in the early part of the decade and for the association – although it was apolitical, most of its members had strong pro-Labour leanings – it augured well.

As widely expected, the country witnessed a change of government in 1964 when Labour, led by Harold Wilson, took over the reins from the Tories. On the night of the general election, quite a few of us stayed up late to watch the results as they were announced on television. By morning, the winds of change had swept Labour into power and we began to dream that the world would be a better place. But it's strange how well Labour works in opposition, but when put in power it becomes even more conservative than the Conservatives.

In those days, colour discrimination was an all too common phenomenon and one of the things the government did was to set up an organisation called the National Council for the Welfare of Commonwealth Immigrants. It was chaired by the Archbishop of Canterbury, Dr Michael Ramsey. I was appointed a member to advise it on matters of health of the ethnic minorities, as it was a subject badly neglected. A number of migrants who had come to Britain from the Indian sub-continent at the time were already suffering from diseases endemic to the region and as such were in need of immediate attention. Their well-being became an issue for the government as well as the local authorities up and down the country.

The council had extremely limited powers and proved pretty ineffective in dealing with ethnic minority issues. The council was, therefore, soon replaced by the Race Relations Board, with the twin objectives of combating discrimination in education, housing and employment on grounds of race and colour, and of organising the ethnic minority communities into active working groups. This was a welcome development, especially for the Afro-Caribbean groups who were its worst victims.

At the same time a number of Councils for Community Relations were established, one in Manchester. The first Race Relations Act was passed and conciliation committees were formed. The purpose behind these measures was to improve the lot of the migrant community which was playing an increasing role in the economic and social life of the country. The role of the conciliation committees was to promote compliance with the Act and to mediate where there was conflict. The committee based in Manchester was called the North-West Conciliation Committee of the Race Relations Board. Its chairman was Mr Neil Pearson, a prominent lawyer. I was one of its members. Part of our job was to go round various establishments, such as hotels and public houses, preaching the gospel of equality so that the migrants from the new Commonwealth immigrants did not become victims of discrimination on the basis of race and colour.

On one mission, I found myself in a pub in Burnley whose landlord had reportedly refused to serve blacks. I entered the place and asked for a soft drink. The landlord smiled and duly served me. I focussed my gaze on him and asked why he served me so readily when he had reportedly refused the custom of some black members of the community. 'You see, you're a doctor,' he told me. It was gratifying to note that in at least one little corner of England doctors were still held in high esteem, high enough to be served a drink even though they were the wrong colour. We had a long chat, the upshot of which was that we never received any complaint against him again.

The pace of activity picked up in the field of race relations. The Race Relations Act was strengthened and our conciliation committee in Manchester became very busy under the chairmanship of Sir Patrick McColl, Clerk of the Lancashire County Council. I was the vice-chairman. In my new role, I had a lot of work to do, a lot of cases to tackle, plenty of paper work to deal with. Shortly afterwards, I was appointed its chairman and I had to attend meetings in Manchester as well as London regularly. During that period I also got involved with the Afro-Caribbean community. After all, we were, along with other sections of the minorities, working towards the same objective – the eradication of racial prejudice from the country. I made many friends belonging to the Afro-Caribbean community.

One day I received a telephone call from Mr Arthur Jackson, chairman of the Jamaican group. He told me about an Indian by the name of Amol Chatterjee who worked as a designer in their office. A hard-working and conscientious man, he was always punctual and seldom took time off. But all of a sudden he had gone AWOL and no one in the office knew what had happened to him. Mr Jackson asked me if, by any chance, he was a relation of mine. He found my namesake's absence a bit baffling, to say the least. I explained to him that Chatterjee was a fairly common Bengali name. Though not quite in the Smiths and Jones category, it came in the second-eleven of Taylors and Browns. The Chatterjee who worked in his office was not related to me, not even distantly, I told him. However, I was concerned about the gentleman's unexplained absence and promised to do everything possible in tracing his whereabouts, so I made a few inquiries, spread the word on the Indian grapevine but all attempts drew a blank. Then, out of the blue, the local police phoned me one afternoon to tell me that they were holding a gentleman by the name of Chatterjee and would I come and assist them.

The story was that Chatterjee had taken a taxi and told the driver to take him to Nottingham where he was going to meet an old friend. The driver obeyed the instructions and went seventy-odd miles to where his passenger had told him he wanted to go. On reaching Nottingham, Chatterjee said he could not remember the address and asked the driver to turn back to Manchester. On arrival back in Manchester, the taxi driver demanded the money, which must have been a large amount, but Chatterjee, instead of paying him in cash, gave him a cheque drawn on a bank in India.

Understandably, tempers must have frayed and the driver took him straight to the nearest police station. The police interrogated the Indian and locked him in a cell where, unable to stand the cold of the place, he set fire to the mattress. Chatterjee was charged by police with arson and moved to Risley Remand Centre. I went to see him there and he looked a desperate man, ill, unshaven and incoherent. He was making no sense at all. I was concerned, for he was a classic case of mental illness. Mentally ill people behave differently from normal people when they are under stress and it was clear that Chatterjee was under great stress. I aired this view to the officers who told me that they would have him seen to by their own doctor.

A few days later I made inquiries about him and was told that he had been tried in Leeds and sent to prison for six months on charges of arson. I was deeply upset, for I thought the man was not in full possession of his faculties and should have been treated rather than jailed. I went to see him in prison and found him in a state of total bewilderment. It was as if he didn't know what was happening to him or to things around him. When I inquired if the prisoner was receiving any psychiatric help, I was told that now that I had brought up the subject the prison authorities would make sure he was seen by a psychiatrist. On examination it was later discovered that he was really mentally ill. But as he had already been sentenced it was thought he should serve his term.

I raised the matter with one of the local MPs, Sir Leslie Lever. I explained the whole case to him. He promised to take up the case with the relevant authorities but he was also of the opinion that, as the case had been adjudicated, there was little he could do. A few days later, Sir Leslie telephoned to tell me he had been able to persuade the Home Secretary to grant the prisoner the Queen's pardon. Chatterjee was released and referred to a psychiatric hospital for treatment.

In the normal course of my working day at the hospital, I was asked one day by Macclesfield General Hospital to have a look at one of their patients. After visiting the hospital, I stopped at a farm shop to pick up some fresh produce. As the shop was out of potatoes at the time, the saleswoman directed me to a warehouse on Lees Lane, Wilmslow, where, she said, they sold five or six varieties of potatoes and the prices were really knockdown. Unable to resist a bargain, I turned the car in the direction of the warehouse. I went inside and was greeted by a man, tall, red-faced and eager to help. He gave me a sack of potatoes for half a crown – a bargain by all accounts worth writing home about. As he was putting the potatoes in the boot of the car he turned to me and, quite unexpectedly, asked if I was a doctor.

'Yes, I'm a doctor,' I replied.

'Could you have a look at my chest, please; I've been having this pain for the past . . .' and he went on to explain the symptoms of his discomfort and supply other details, such as age and name.

I listened to him patiently and then said, 'Yes, Mr Park, I'm a doctor but I don't practise kerbside medicine. Here's my card. If you want me to see you professionally, please come to see me at Baguley Hospital where I work.'

'All right, doctor,' he said smilingly, understanding my position. 'I'll see you in the hospital.'

'And, yes,' I added as an afterthought, 'do bring a note from your family doctor.'

'OK, doctor, a note from my GP,' he nodded.

I came away happy in the knowledge that I had enough potatoes to last the family at least a month and the whole lot of them had cost me a pittance. About three weeks later I was busy in my office with one thing or another when my secretary informed me there was a gentleman to see me.

'But I've no appointment in my diary this morning,' I said somewhat crossly to her, implying that she should have dealt with the person herself.

'He says you asked him to see you in hospital,' she returned.

'All right, let him in,' I said.

A few seconds later in walked Mr Park, Ernie Park, whose potatoes I had been eating almost daily for three weeks in every conceivable form, boiled, fried, mashed, baked, roasted and sautéd. I examined him, assured him there was nothing seriously wrong, gave him a date for a fortnight later to come again and shook hands with him. That handshake marked the start of a friendship that lasted until his death just a few years ago. He had appointed me as his family doctor, paid or unpaid, and I was the first to hear if there was any medical problem in the family. Kind, generous and pleasant, he was one of the nicest people I've met in my life. I greatly value those years of friendship with Ernie Park. And, I'm glad to say, we are still friends of the family.

CHAPTER 11

Return to India

LIFE CAN BE FULL of surprises and the odd, occasional shock. It came as I was visiting my friend Sardar Bahadur one evening. As the door opened for me, tension hung in the air like pollen on a hot summer's afternoon. Sardar, his wife and their nephew were locked in a heated and bitter argument. I sat in the lounge while they, in another room well out of my sight, tried to come to an amicable agreement or postpone the discussion to some other time. At the heart of the argument lay the nephew's association with a certain young woman. Things had apparently gone pretty far, so far in fact that he had expressed the desire to marry her, something of which Sardar strongly disapproved. Somewhere between these two polar positions was the view Mrs Bahadur held. As I sat there casually flicking through the newspaper, Sardar, being the head of the family, decided to call time on the subject and sent the two of them to attend to their restaurant and the evening customers. As they left, he told me he was going to have a lie-down for about half an hour. I could, in the meantime, read something or watch television or whatever. So off he went upstairs for a rest while I continued to keep myself busy with the paper.

Suddenly there was a sound of commotion and Sardar shouted to me to come upstairs and help him as he was feeling terribly unwell. I rushed to where he was and found that he was having a heart attack. As it was difficult for one person to manage him single-handed, I immediately telephoned for an ambulance. It responded with amazing speed, for barely had I put the telephone down when I could see its flashing lights through the window. As Sardar, wrapped in a blanket, was being eased into the ambulance, I telephoned the restaurant to inform his wife and to let her know that I was going to Baguley Hospital where he was being taken. Sadly, the attack was a massive one and he was pronounced dead on arrival. He was a very close friend and his death left a huge gap in our lives.

At Baguley Hospital, my workload was increasing at an amazing pace. The laboratory I had set up was successful and we were being taken note of by medical organisations in Britain as well as in India. The hospital's tuberculosis unit had changed to a chest unit and it was also undertaking research and investigation into other chest diseases, such as bronchitis and asthma. At the same time a number of pharmaceutical companies wanted us to try out their new drugs for treatment of these diseases. In addition I was again getting a number of invitations from Delhi, Bombay, Calcutta and other major cities in India to give a series of lectures on the work my unit was doing. This time, however, my mind was made up that if I decided to go to the sub-continent I'd take my family with me so that they could have their first taste of India.

Our two daughters, Camille and Petula, were growing up and busy with their studies so they were not able to come with us. They were doing well at Fylde Lodge School and Withington High respectively and were at a stage where they could not take nearly a month off during term time. Our son Nigel, who was at Stockport Grammar Prep Department, was given permission to accompany us. Having all three of our children attending grammar schools was really heavy on the pocket but at the same time it was so satisfying to see what they were making of their lives. Both girls were in their teens and keen to take care of themselves while we were away. We were wondering what we should do when our neighbouring family pleasantly surprised us by offering to take them under their wing during the period we were away. My wife Enid was still worried about them but repeated assurances from our neighbour prevailed on her.

So, one fine morning, Enid, Nigel (armed with homework and a project) and myself set off for London for the onward flight to Bombay. At Santa Cruz airport, we were met by Dr Gopal Ghatikar, who very kindly offered to take us to our hotel. My lectures were well received and our stay in Bombay was a thoroughly enjoyable one. We were treated to excellent hospitality by the city's medical fraternity. While in Bombay, I decided to take the family to Kanniyakumari, which is the southernmost tip of India. I had always wanted to go there but one thing or another somehow got in the way and I couldn't make it during my time as a medical student or while serving in the army. Now I had time as well as the means and I wasn't going to let the opportunity slip through my fingers.

Hindu mythology is full of legends and Kanniyakumari is not without one. In the Hindu triumvirate there are three lords: Brahma the creator, Vishnu the preserver and Shiva the destroyer. The legend has it that when Lord Shiva reached marriageable age, Parvati, one of the goddesses, had a crush on him and wanted to marry him. She made her intentions known to him but he fought off her amorous advances. Things came to such a pass that she started stalking him. To escape from her, he decided to leave his Himalayan abode in the north and go as far away as he could. Off he went to the end of the land some 3,000 miles away until he could go no further because of the sea. There he sat down on a rock and tried to lose himself in meditation. But, undeterred, she came in hot pursuit of him and caught up with him. They got married in Kanniyakumari and later returned to the Himalayas as god and wife. It is said that the imprints of her feet can still be seen on one of the rocks. I had known of the legend since my boyhood days but what a thrill it was being where all this romantic drama is supposed to have taken place. Kanniyakumari is where the Indian Ocean, the Arabian Sea and the Bay of Bengal meet. It's truly a wonderful experience to sit on the rock in the evenings and watch nature put on its most spectacular display, the sun falling headlong into restless waves, dramatic in its gold, pink and purple flames, the fish leaping into the air as if trying to catch some of the sun's molten gold.

From Kanniyakumari we flew to Delhi to the stark reality of work. Waiting for us at Palam Airport was Shanta Bhargava, with a huge welcoming smile on her face. With great warmth, she greeted Enid and Nigel and then all four of us piled into a taxi and headed for Bhagwandas Road where the Bhargavas lived and where we were given another hearty welcome, this time from the rest of the members of the family. After a day's rest I delivered my lecture to the Delhi doctors on bronchial asthma. With my only official engagement in the city out of the way we went gallivanting round Delhi, taking in the sights – the Red Fort, Quatab Minar, India Gate and the rest.

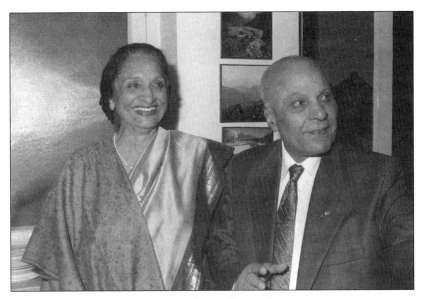

The author with Dr Shanta Bhargava

Shanta and her husband Kamta were keen that we should also visit the Taj Mahal, just over 100 miles away in Agra. I, too, wanted Enid and Nigel to see this great monument, described by Nobel laureate Rabindranath Tagore as 'a teardrop in marble'. Early one morning a taxi arrived on our doorstep to take us to the Taj. Inspired by his love for his wife Mumtaz, the Moghul Emperor Shah Jahan built it some 350 years ago to enshrine her body. The Taj enjoys the reputation of being one of the wonders of the modern world and it is not difficult to see why. A World Heritage site now, the monument never disappoints those who come to Agra from all over the world to see a man-made masterpiece. Shimmering white in its majesty during the day, the Taj presents an altogether different picture at night. We had seen it in daylight so it was agreed that we should also see it in moonlight. The cool sparkle of marble is very soothing at that hour and has a calming effect on the soul. Small wonder then that, night or day, for centuries, poets have stood in its shadows thinking and writing about their own love.

From Agra we returned to Delhi. Barely had we rested for a few hours when Shanta suggested that we should also take in some Hindu holy sites, as it would be a novel experience for Enid and Nigel on their maiden visit to India. Kamta's sister, Sheela Bhargava, professor of anaesthetics at Delhi Medical College, and her husband, Satyanand Kumar, professor of surgery at the same institution, also joined us and during our travels we became good friends with them.

The holy city of Haridwar is not very far from Delhi. There are also other attractions near by, like Rishikesh and Laxman Jhula, a rickety rope bridge over the River Ganges and straddling two mountains. It really is a sight to see and, once you've been on it, an experience to remember. We arrived at Haridwar and Shanta proposed that my wife should have a bath in the Ganges because, according to popular myth, a dip in this holy river washes away a person's sins. Eager to 'cleanse' themselves, our two Indian hostesses and my wife went to the changing rooms, wrapped themselves in cotton saris, drew a deep breath and plunged into the freezing water.

Another popular custom for those visiting Haridwar is that, after a bath in the river, they do a *pooja* ceremony – a chanting of prayers – on the riverbank and, as an act of charity, distribute cooked food to the holy men, the poor and the destitute. Following current customs, we gave money to one of the 'providers' who, within a matter of minutes, conjured up hundreds of *puris* – a kind of fried pancake – and two or three cooked vegetables to go as accompaniments. Holding piles of *puris* in their hands, the three women started distributing them among the poor on a green. When they began, there was hardly a soul in sight but word must have spread on the grapevine because suddenly out of nowhere hordes of beggars and saffron-clad sadhus appeared and a stampede for food started. For a time there was complete mayhem and at one stage the situation got so out of control that the three of them had to be 'rescued' by their husbands from hungry hands demanding food.

We returned from Haridwar exhausted and carrying a bruised conscience over the poverty which we had just witnessed. It was now time to begin the final leg of our Indian journey. It took us to my home town of Patna, where, for the first time, Enid and Nigel met other members of our family. We then moved on to

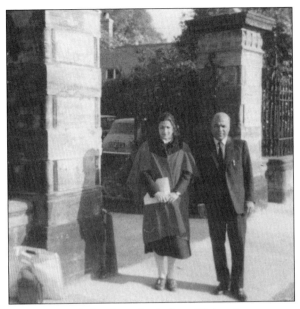

With Petula at St Andrews University

Calcutta where I delivered my final lecture, which was well received by the medical fraternity of the city. And then, once again, England was on our minds. Though the whole trip was overshadowed by bouts of Delhi belly, Bombay tummy and what have you, it was nevertheless a thoroughly enjoyable experience. We made new friends, cemented old relationships and were happy with the memories we brought back to Manchester to share with our daughters.

As time wore on, Camille passed her A-level examinations and expressed the desire to go into nursing and Pet decided that she would like to study medicine. I was delighted with their choice of such purposeful professions. In early 1968, Camille joined Radcliffe Infirmary in Oxford where she was to spend the next three and a half years. Pet, on the other hand, took up medicine at St Andrews University. We were pleased with her choice because medical students at St Andrews spend a sizeable chunk of their time in Manchester hospitals. This meant that she would be with us although her university was in Scotland. We promised both girls a car each and soon they were behind the steering wheels of their own vehicles.

CHAPTER 12

Recognition

BARRING THE ODD INCIDENT or two, the second trip to India was as enjoyable as the first one – in many ways more so because I had my wife and son for company. By undertaking to give lectures in far-flung corners of India I was, in a way, promoting closer co-operation between the medical institutions of the two countries and also clearing the path for more such visits in the future – not only by myself but also by other doctors from Britain. Going to another country to meet and speak to highly qualified doctors and academics at some of the best institutions in the country is not as simple as it seems on the surface A lot of preparatory work has to be done beforehand. Sometimes it can takes weeks of research to prepare a lecture that is over in less than an hour. But I think the effort is worth it in the end. After all, the ultimate aim of medicine and of those who practise it is to eliminate human suffering, and an exchange of knowledge goes a long way towards that end.

After a few hours' rest on my return from India I was, as they say, back in the old routine – hospital work, research work, publications, the occasional lecture here and there. Soon I felt that all these activities were showing a significant rise. While I was assessing and reassessing the situation, I received a telephone call from Geoffrey Jessop, inviting me to a Rotary Club lunch. Always keen on lunch, especially when invited, I accepted the offer with alacrity, thinking I'd squeeze the lunch between my morning and afternoon sessions at work.

About thirty or so people sat round a number of tables in the hotel where the meeting had been arranged. From what I could gather they were mainly talking about themselves and their work for the club. A three-course lunch soon followed, after which the guest speaker had his turn. It was all new to me but I found it quite interesting. While busy with the lunch, I wondered why I had been invited to it but I soon discovered that the club wanted me to join up. In other words, it was a sort of vetting exercise which I had no doubt I had passed with flying colours. A young, smart and amiable member of the branch came and sat next to me. With a huge grin on his face, he extended his hand in my direction and introduced himself as Ron Anderson. With that friendly shake of hands, we became close and personal friends. I had always admired the work the Rotarians did all over the world and so, within days of that luncheon meeting, I joined the movement.

I was soon to discover that while all clubs did marvellous charitable work, ours was rather well stocked in the ambition department. It wanted to do things, go places, produce results. In one particular project, it joined forces with another club to send equipment to Seranga Hospital in a relatively poor area of West Bengal. Our club had decided that it would provide electricity and power equipment to the hospital. I thought it was a case where I could be helpful and soon I found myself getting in touch with the Indian High Commission in London, discussing plans to transport a transformer to the hospital so that it could have its own source of power supply.

I must admit that, in those days, negotiating the purchase of a transformer and then having it shipped to India was a subject millions of miles from my street. It still is. Strangely enough, Enid had contacts at the time with a Methodist mission in Manchester. They informed her that the P&O shipping line reserved for charities a small percentage of the freight that it moved. We immediately laid claim to a small part of that small part. The Calcutta Rotary Club and the West Bengal government offered to help in speeding up the bureaucratic processes by cutting out some of the red tape and also to negotiate us through the rest.

As preparations were going on for shipping the transformer, I noticed on my way from one part of Baguley Hospital to another a number of old iron bedsteads stacked up in a corner, seemingly headed for the tip. Coming from a background where nothing is wasted if it has an ounce of utility left in it, the sight of those beds rang a bell: these beds would do nicely in the hospital where our transformer was going to light up the wards. All that the beds needed was a lick of paint here and a spit and polish there and

Seranga could be our double beneficiary. So at the first chance I arranged to meet our hospital's treasurer, Mr Geoff Pearson, and went straight to the point, without any preamble.

'Are those bedsteads destined for the scrap heap, Geoff?' I asked.

'Certainly not,' he answered. 'Whatever gave you that idea?'

'It's just the way they're kept, in a haphazard fashion, neglected, as if they've outlived their usefulness.'

'Oh, I see. The reason why they're kept that way is because they're not going to be used here. They're for sale.'

'For sale?' I gasped. 'I don't believe it. Who'll buy that useless lot?'

'You want to make an offer?'

'I don't think I can. I haven't got that kind of money.'

'What kind of money are we talking about?'

'I don't know, Geoff. I honestly don't.'

'You can have the lot for £10 if you want. Now does that sound excessive to you? Surely, you've got that kind of money.'

'Well, I don't know, a bit exorbitant,' I smiled. 'But here's the cheque.'

We shook hands and with that 120 iron bedsteads changed hands for £10. The cheque was his and the beds were mine. But the snag was that I didn't have a clue what to do with them except that I wanted them to go to the Indian hospital where they could be put to good use. Faced with the prospect of having to shift 120 beds from one hospital to another 5,000 miles away without the foggiest idea how to go about it, I approached my trusted friend, mentor and guide, Ron Anderson. Ever eager to oblige, he made it sound as if there was no problem at all.

'I shall have a word with Jack and his wife Ruth,' he enthused. 'They have a shop in Sharston and I'm sure they'll have storage space for them for a few days.'

Storage pace for the beds they did have, and the generous couple offered it to us gladly. The beds were moved to Jack and Ruth's shop and stored above it. Jack and Ruth carried the dismantled rods upstairs themselves. We also found a painter to give the irons a lick of shine so they would look quite presentable when they reached their final destination in West Bengal. A year later I visited Seranga and it was undiluted joy to see – thanks to the efforts of a bunch of selfless, dedicated Rotarians in Manchester – the brightly-lit wards and corridors of the hospital that also boasted 'imported' beds for its patients.

Round about this time I received a letter from the Royal College of Physicians of Edinburgh. They had decided to offer me the membership of the college without an examination. It's a dream come true for any youngish doctor to have MRCP to add to his or her name and a lot of medics would give their right arm to get the membership *with* an exam. I went to Edinburgh and was warmly greeted by the president of the college. We had lunch and following that I met members of the college council. They asked me if the offer was acceptable to me. Acceptable? I was ready to snatch it from their hands. In the conversation with them I could detect unmistakable hints that the college would like to confer on me fellowship at some later stage. I wasn't wrong in my guesswork for in the following year I was once again beating a track to Edinburgh – this time to be made a fellow.

One thing surprised, though. Here was the Royal College of Physicians of Edinburgh ready and willing to bestow on me the honour of an exam-free fellowship while the Royal College of Physicians of London, of which I had been a member for a number of years, had conveniently chosen to look the other way. There was this perceived notion among many doctors, especially from overseas, that the London college was at best slow in recognising the ability and achievements of foreign-trained doctors and at worst it was discriminatory. It was the experience of many overseas medics who had passed their membership exam that it usually took them longer to get their fellowship than the home-grown variety. However, soon enough I did receive a letter from London offering me fellowship of the college.

So here I was with the most basic medical qualification when I arrived in Britain a couple of decades before, now a Fellow of the Royal College of Physicians of Edinburgh, as well as of the Royal College of Physicians of London. Boy, did I feel glad about it? You bet I did. I was on a high, which was very high. Then, just as the descent to earth was gradually beginning, a letter arrived in the morning post from Manchester magistrates' court, its chairman informing me I had been selected as a magistrate for the city of Manchester. He wanted me to arrange a meeting with the secretary to discuss details. I did not know what it meant to be a magistrate but I was certainly aware that it was something of great importance and had to be taken seriously. I accepted the offer and after a few days was handling my first case as a magistrate, one of the first, if not the first, magistrate of Indian origin to sit in a court.

Among the first cases I dealt with was one concerning a scrawny slip of a girl. She was before the court on charges of 'loitering with intent'. I was wondering what intent an under-nourished girl who seemed barely into her teens would have when someone whispered in my ear that she was a prostitute and was loitering with the intention of picking up clients. As the case gradually unfolded, it was revealed that she was single, had no home to live in and no money to live on. After both sides had put forward their arguments and a decision was reached she was found guilty and I decided to fine her £2. To me that seemed quite reasonable. On hearing the verdict, she turned her pockets inside out and held out a sixpence to show to the court. That's all she had in the whole wide world. It was clear that she was in no position to pay the fine. As chairman of the magistrates that day what was I supposed to do next? I looked at the clerk of the court who understood the position well. We went into a huddle behind the chairs and it was agreed that if she changed her plea to guilty the court would give her a conditional discharge. She did and we discharged her conditionally. She walked out of the court with her sixpence still in tact and I was relieved I didn't have to put the girl, who didn't even have two coins to rub together, under greater financial strain.

Early one morning I was having breakfast, when a letter arrived. It was addressed to me and marked 'Confidential' in bold letters. On one corner of the envelope were the words: 'From the Prime Minister'. I looked at it carefully and then looked again with even greater care, playing a secret, guessing game with myself over what it might contain. The morning had certainly given me more than breakfast to chew. I fidgeted with the letter for a few moments and then, before opening it, showed it to Enid. 'It says here "From the Prime Minister",' I said to her between a bite and a swallow.

'I think it's got your deportation order,' she quipped and giggled. Mildly, I laughed, too. The thought going through my mind was that I could do with a few days of inactivity, watching from my deportation camp window a herd of Friesians, heads bowed, happily grazing in the field, in the background ripening corn swaying in the breeze. The hectic lifestyle had left no time for these simple pleasures. Rest, indolence, free time? Ah, what bliss! But, ah, what wishful thinking!

Yes, the letter was indeed from the Prime Minister. It said he intended honouring me with a civil award. It then went on to explain, if the honour was acceptable to me, how to proceed with the formalities and the paperwork involved. I didn't expect in my wildest dreams to be honoured with an OBE. From the mists of outer space in which I was then floating, cloud nine seemed no more than a tiny speck. And this remained my state of mind for the next few days. Along with the letter was an acceptance form which had to be filled in and returned. I took the letter to the hospital with me that morning and gave it to my secretary, Mrs Laura Dennison. As she read it, her hands began to tremble and, when she had read it a second time, she began to cry. Tears of joy, I presumed. She was, she said, overwhelmed. She had never touched a letter from so important a person as the Prime Minister of Great Britain. I said something funny to stop the flow of her tears and told her, before she soaked the letter with her tears, to type my reply and put it in the post. This she did as the next thing that morning. After a few days I received another letter giving me a date to come to London to receive my OBE.

It was a glorious morning in London in more ways than one for me. The sun was beating down as, accompanied by Enid, our elder daughter Camille and son Nigel, I made my way to Buckingham Palace. Each of us was decked in brand new clothes and shoes that had not a single speck of dust on them. A lot of planning had gone into who would wear what for, after all, we were going to London to meet the Queen. My friend from Patna Medical College, Dr Sunil Bhattacharya, who was a GP in

London, had offered to chauffeur us to the Palace as a special treat for us. We went through the entry procedure. Then I was separated from my family and taken to an area from where I was ushered in to receive my OBE from Her Majesty the Queen. It was indeed an honour. There I was, shaking hands with the Queen, having my medal pinned on my chest by her. I was filled with pride. I was proud of myself, proud of my achievements, proud of being a doctor in Britain. Life was indeed on a roll. In the past three years or so I had become a consultant, a fellow of two Royal Colleges, a magistrate and now a proud Officer of the British Empire.

One morning, I received a telephone call. It was a student, Tom Bailey, at the other end in Coventry. He told me he had been advised by somebody to get in touch with me on a rather private matter. Having digested that, I expected him next to reel out the symptoms of his malady, but he didn't.

'Yes, Tom, get in touch with me, but why?' I politely asked. 'What have I done?'

'Well, actually it's not what you've done but what you can do.'

It was quite flattering to hear that in some quarters of the community I was considered a can-do man.

'Fire away, dear fellow,' I answered. 'If I can do it then consider it done.'

'It's a matter of a rather personal nature and instead of talking on the phone I'd like to discuss it with you in person. Is that all right?'

'Of course it is,' I assured him. 'Come next Saturday morning, if you're free, and we can have a chat.'

'Fine, just fine. See you on Saturday then.' The meeting arranged, he put the phone down.

I soon got busy with my work at the hospital and other things that I had in plenty. Saturday morning came and with it a knock on the front door. As I opened it, standing before me with a smile on his face was Tom Bailey, tall, handsome and fresh-faced. A couple of feet behind him stood an Indian girl to whom I was quickly introduced by Tom. She was Manjit, his girl friend and a fellow-student with him in Coventry. I led them into the lounge and we settled down with a cup of tea.

'Manjit and I have been studying at Coventry Polytechnic for the past three years,' Tom began. 'We've been friends . . . more than friends, really, and now we want to get married.'

'Good, good,' I said enthusiastically. 'When is the big day?'

'That's the problem . . . or rather Manjit's dad is the problem. He is dead against it and threatened that if I got married to her he'd kill me.'

'Oh dear,' I gasped. 'You do have a serious problem, young man.'

'Not only that,' Tom added rather sheepishly. 'I told him I was going to seek your advice and he said that he'd kill you also.'

'Oh dear,' I said with a hand on my heart, 'it seems I've a serious problem too. But tell me, why would he come all the way from Coventry to kill me?'

As if on cue, the telephone rang and the man with double murder on his mind in order to 'protect' his nubile daughter from a white man and a counselling doctor spoke.

'My name is Kirpal Singh and my daughter and a white boy are with you at this moment,' he said in a serious, almost solemn, tone. 'There's no use denying it because I know they are.'

'I'm not denying it,' I answered. 'Yes, the two of them are here with me this minute. We're having a discussion.'

'What's there to discuss?' After that he prattled on in Hindi and Punjabi for a while, the gist of which was that if the two of them decided to do something rash and against his wishes, he would soon be on his way to put an end to all that.

I wasn't really worried but I must admit I was definitely concerned. Holding the receiver in one hand, I listened patiently to his tirade, my mind quietly taking stock of the serious situation. A few yards away from me in the lounge sat an Indian girl, a complete stranger until that morning, crying her heart out. Opposite her was her white boyfriend, also a stranger, with a death threat hanging over his head and here I was with an irate father after my blood in a scenario that wasn't of my making.

In a placatory voice that demanded reason, I said to the angry caller from Coventry, 'Mr Singh, I'd like to meet you.' That, he replied, would only hasten the contact between his dagger and my body. I repeated my offer to meet him, adding, 'Look, trust me

I'm a doctor, Mr Singh,' – the implication being that I was an educated person, perfectly capable of reasoning things out and bringing about an amicable settlement in the dispute – 'I've your daughter in my house and also the young man. They both look nice young people who are in love with each other. Why don't you let them marry?'

'Let them get married? And what about my *izzat*, my honour?'

'I know your honour is important, but you've got to balance it against the life-long happiness of your daughter.'

'No, my life would be ruined.' He repeated this three or four times.

However, by the end of the conversation, he had offered to put the death sentences on Tom and myself on hold for a few days. Immensely relieved, I rejoined the young couple with an uneasy smile. Then I signed a cheque for £50 and gave it to Tom and Manjit as my contribution towards their honeymoon and told them to go to Didsbury and see Roy Allison, a young priest and a personal friend, who would help them plan their wedding.

It all ended happily as, a few days later, Tom got his girl and the girl got her man. Tom's mother was pleased that her son was unscathed and I was pleased that no steel dagger had penetrated my heart. A few months later I received an invitation for a meal – from Kirpal Singh of Coventry. I didn't know whether to accept it or not. Maybe he had had a complete change of heart or maybe he thought poisoning was a better method to get rid of interfering doctors. But as I have complete faith in the generosity of the human spirit, I accepted. A few days later Enid and I were on our way to meet the Singh clan. We were greeted with great warmth. The family lived in a good house. An excellent spread was laid out for us – good food, good conversation and, surprise, surprise, sharing all this with was young Tom. Not only was he one of the family but he had become the manager of Mr Singh's taxi firm. Three cheers for love's triumph over odds!

While busy with my clinic at the hospital one afternoon, I received a telephone call from David Harris, medical director of a pharmaceutical company in London. He wanted to come and see me about a new drug that his company was working on. The idea was to try the drug on some of my severely asthmatic patients as I had a large number of them. Promising nothing, I agreed to see him and a date was fixed. On the appointed date he arrived at Baguley Hospital with another doctor. Both of them went into details of their aerosol steroids which they wanted to try on my cases. After listening to them attentively, I developed some doubts over their new drug. Aerosol steroids had been tried before and had not produced any spectacular results. The two went away seemingly a little disappointed with my response.

That, however, wasn't the end of the story. A few days later, Dr Harris was back again in Manchester. A lengthy discussion ensued and because of the faith he showed in the drug and the fact that trials of the drug were being conducted at some London hospitals, I relented, on condition that I would first seek the approval of my medical ethics committee and only after they had given the go-ahead would the drug be tried on my patients. In due course I saw the chairman of the committee, Dr Les Doyle, and explained the whole situation to him. He agreed to submit my application to the committee and, following their meeting, permission was granted. Trials began at Baguley and proved a resounding success. We now had the answer to the problems of asthma patients in the shape of aerosol steroids. The trials were among the earliest in the field and I was glad that, in my own small way, I was instrumental in the success of aerosol steroids.

CHAPTER 13

The Overseas Doctors' Association

MY DAUGHTER CAMILLE, who had gone to Oxford to do nursing training, was coming towards the end of her three-year course. She called home one evening and invited us for a meal. All that way for a meal? That was my initial reaction when I first heard about it. I thought there was more to the lunch or dinner than met the eye. But since we had not seen her for a while, we decided to accept her invitation and go to Oxford to meet and eat with her. We set off from Manchester in the morning and reached Oxford in the early afternoon. Our destination was Radcliffe Infirmary, where she was training. We collected her from her hostel and headed for a riverside restaurant. It was a bright, sunny afternoon and, as we were flicking through the tasselled menu, a young man, wearing a smart, casual outfit and with a slightly nervous smile pasted on his face, walked in and came to a halt near our table. Camille introduced him to us as Paul Periton. I motioned him to a chair and he joined us for lunch. Paul, a graduate from Cambridge, was studying for his master's degree in economics at Oxford, where the two of them had come into contact with each other.

The meal was a thoroughly enjoyable affair, the conversation equally delightful. We chatted about this and that and about the many big and small things in life that we all have in common. I liked Paul. He was polite, decent and idealistic. The meal over, we parted company and, shortly after that, my wife and I set off back to Manchester. The thoughts that go through the minds of fathers with daughters of marriageable age had recently been preying on my mind, too. Driving back, I kept thinking about my daughter and what she would do once she had qualified as a nurse. Would she live in Oxford or move somewhere else? How would Paul figure in her future plans?

A few days later my wife informed me that we were going to have a visit from our daughter and her boyfriend. Welcome

118

home, Camille! On the agreed day the two of them arrived and started fussing over me and wanting to take me out for a meal along with the rest of the family. My suspicious mind wondered what had made them come all the way to Manchester from Oxford, make me the focal point of their attention and want to give me a treat at a restaurant of my own choosing. Ah, well, well, something was definitely up. I didn't have to endure the suspense for long, because soon Paul came into the garden where he found me momentarily alone and asked to have a word with me if it was all right. Of course it was all right.

'Go right ahead,' I said to him, and waited. After some hesitant pauses and tentative throat clearing, he told me that he wanted the hand of my daughter in marriage. I was half-expecting something of that nature. Focussing my eyes on him, I studied his face carefully. It wasn't the pleasantly surprising nature of his question that had engaged my attention but the fact that, in the fast changing values of the sixties and the early seventies, here was a young man who was courteous enough to seek my permission to marry my daughter. As far as I was concerned I couldn't have found a better person myself if I had gone out looking for one, but had he spoken to his would-be mother-in-law? He hadn't because he thought he would start with me. Perhaps he was expecting that I would be the hardest nut to crack in the family. I went inside and asked my wife where Camille was. She informed me that she was upstairs in the bedroom, busy with one thing or another. Just then, as in a stage play, she made an appearance on the landing. She stood there for a few seconds and then started to come down the stairs slowly, wiping her moist eyes with a Kleenex. Apparently, she had been in the bathroom and not the bedroom, crying her eyes out in case I objected to the marriage plan and refused to give my permission. Worse still, she feared I would have her packed off to India to find a suitable boy in an arranged marriage safari. When she told me all this, I found it both amazing and amusing. I assured her that the thought had never crossed my mind. Not even once. I told her that I had had a long chat with her intended and given him the go-ahead and my blessings and I was pleased for them both. The tension in the house – if it was there I wasn't even aware of it let alone being

a party to it – evaporated. There were cackles of laughter and
doubtless a few tears of joy were shed in secret corners. It was
then agreed that we would all go out for a meal and –
call it excitement or carelessness – I offered to pay the bill.

It was a good and extremely pleasant family occasion and
included in it was my future son-in-law, who was soon to
complete his degree from Oxford and take up a job as a lecturer
in Nottingham. He would move to the city in the near future.
Camille also said she'd like to work in Nottingham. We had a
long chat and it was agreed that she'd get married on 9 September
1972. The Dean of Manchester Cathedral, Alfred Jowett, was a
friend of mine and, when he heard about Camille's plan to get
married, he offered to perform the ceremony if the marriage were
to take place in Manchester. But Paul and Camille had other
ideas. Paul had a friend in Plymouth who had just joined the
ecclesiastical service and he decided to have him for the service.
I sent out invitations to a number of my Indian friends in
Manchester but had my doubts about anyone turning up in
Plymouth for the ceremony because of the distance. But I had
underestimated their enthusiasm, for when we arrived at the
church on the wedding day I was amazed and delighted to find
sixteen couples from Manchester ready and waiting to share in
our joy. All of them were there and what a wonderful wedding
gift their presence was to our family. A reception was held after
the ceremony and a week later I arranged a big function in
Manchester, which was attended by more than 600 people.

My wife and I were pleased that our elder daughter was now
happily married and going to settle not very far from us. Petula
was by now a third-year medical student and she was back in
Manchester to do her clinical part. She got herself a flat in
Didsbury which she shared with fellow-student Cathy O'Flynn.
Our son Nigel, meanwhile, continued his studies at Stockport
Grammar.

While things were chugging alone nicely on the domestic
front, I received a letter from Dr Akram Sayeed, a general
practitioner who had come to Britain from Bangladesh and built
up a busy practice in Leicester. The purpose of his letter was to
draw attention to the plight of young overseas doctors working in

Britain. I had also noticed that the medical press, along with the tabloid section of the mainstream press, was taking an increasingly hostile attitude towards the overseas doctors in its coverage and portrayed them in a very bad light, as if all the ills of the National Health Service were of their making. The number of doctors coming to the United Kingdom from the Indian subcontinent was doubtless on the increase. Among them were graduates more or less straight out of universities and medical colleges with no experience to speak of. Many of them were finding themselves in jobs for which they were neither trained nor suited. Then there were those who were either overqualified or underqualified. In short, too many square pegs in round holes. The upshot of all this was that there was a lot of dissatisfaction among new arrivals and that dissatisfaction in turn created new problems. And as doctors who were dealing with lives of people, their problems had to be tackled head on and resolved.

The general perception among Britain's overseas medical community was that the criticism levelled against them was grossly unfair. Many doctors who had come to Britain had training in disciplines for which there were no jobs in this country and so they found themselves working in specialities for which they had not been adequately trained. In a number of cases, those specialised in medicine ended up working in orthopaedics, while those seeking positions in obstetrics and gynaecology ended up examining ears, noses and throats. From the point of view of overseas doctors, I felt that they were being used as just an extra pair of hands and that their career aspirations were ignored.

Dr Sayeed's letter worked as a spur to do something to remedy the situation. I was also aware that if I got involved with the problems of overseas doctors it might have an adverse effect on my future advancement. Even though I was a senior consultant, there were areas for further advancement. After a lot of deliberations and soul-searching, however, I decided to put caution in my back pocket and work towards forming a body which would look after the interests of young overseas doctors. So on May 12, 1976 a meeting was held at the home of Dr S. Venogopal, an Indian GP from Aston, Birmingham, at which about twenty doctors were present. An ad hoc committee was set up with the express aim of taking the movement forward. I was chosen as the vice-president. We also decided, as a way to gauge the temperature of feelings, to visit hospitals up and down the country and talk to as many overseas doctors working there as possible and listen to their problems. We went to a number of hospitals and what we already knew was confirmed in one meeting after another with them. Within no time it was clear to us that there was a desperate need for an association.

About four months later, the first conference of overseas doctors was held in London on September 19, 1976. It was attended by more than 120 doctors. Dr Venogopal, Dr Admani and Dr Sayeed played important roles in the formation of the Overseas Doctors' Association – ODA. On the day of the meeting, I also had to go to a hospital in London where my friend, Dr Sunil Bhattacharya – he was the one who had driven us to Buckingham Palace on my investiture day – was recovering from a heart bypass operation. I went into the room where he was alone. I felt sorry for him. He was away from home, had undergone major heart surgery and had no one to look after him in his hour of need. I sat with him for a time, held his hand and we conversed for some time about the good old days when we were medical students in Patna and how we had come to Britain and all that. After visiting him, I returned to the conference hotel and was greeted with cries of enthusiastic congratulations and back-slapping. Congratulations for what? I was soon to discover that in my absence they had voted me overwhelmingly as the chairman of the newly-formed body. Chairman of ODA? But I didn't know the first thing about running a professional association. I couldn't work out what to make of my new role. I had no experience of any kind and at any level in the field, no team to help and assist me, no strategy to follow. Just loads and loads of other people's problems.

But I was also aware that somewhere in this massively confusing picture lay a challenge, and a challenge I always find hard to resist. So I made up my mind that I'd have a jolly good crack at it. Mentally I gave myself five years in which to resolve these problems, even if it meant putting my future professional advancement at risk. I felt it was important that doctors coming from abroad should be provided with proper training facilities, where training was needed, to enable them to carry out their work to the standard expected of them, while at the same time there should be a job structure in place so that they could take their careers forward. The medical establishment at the time had plenty of racial prejudice in its backyard and it hurt to see young, bright overseas doctors become its victims.

But as far as the newly-formed association was concerned, the task it faced looked very daunting. There seemed few highs and numerous lows. Apart from other problems, we had no office, no funds and only limited membership. However, on the bright side I knew the executives of a number of pharmaceutical companies and was sure in my mind that they would help us out if we approached them for assistance. So I made up my mind to tap into that seam. Two of them, Drs Patrick Knowlson and David Harris, I found especially sympathetic to our cause. Dr Harris, who was already helping me in my research work, gave me a cheque for £10,000. I was deeply moved by his generous gesture. That it was a substantial amount there was little doubt. But the value of this large amount to our morale was immeasurable. I telephoned my friend, Dr Admani, and told him that the wagon was ready to roll and that we should keep the momentum going by acquiring, without further loss of time, a place of our own. It's amazing how catching success can be at times. Dr Admani launched his own drive for funds and had within no time raised a large amount himself. Other fund-raising events also brought in varying amounts of money. We now had enough money to set up an office in Manchester's St Peter's Square and were firmly in the business of improving the lot of Britain's overseas doctors and, in turn, providing better service to National Health patients.

June White, already experienced in hospital work, took over the running of the office and what an invaluable asset she proved to be. Although not well-versed in Indian names and surnames – and some of them can be real tongue-twisters at times – she took it upon herself to learn more about them and also about the way some doctors expressed themselves, more directly, less diplomatically. The office was soon a beehive of activity and a venue for regular meetings. Branches of ODA also began to

spring up all over the country, from Leeds to London and from
Burnley to Bristol. This rapid growth phenomenon came as no
surprise to us because by now there were more than 20,000
overseas doctors working in the country.

It was only natural that such a positive response did not go
down well in certain medical establishments. This was only to be
expected, as they saw us as some sort of rebellious, breakaway
group who did not want to be in the British medical mainstream.
This certainly was not true. Young overseas doctors had genuine
grievances and they wanted to give vent to their feelings and saw
ODA as their own vehicle, their collective voice, and one that
would help them secure a fairer deal. Around that time, I wrote
a letter to the British Medical Association and their secretary, Dr
Derek Stevenson, agreed to see a delegation from ODA.

It was a strange meeting, by no means hostile but certainly far
from friendly. There were three of us from ODA – Drs
Venogopal and Admani were the other two – sitting on one side
of a large, rectangular table while members of the BMA sat on
the opposite side. The meeting started on a terse note. Dr

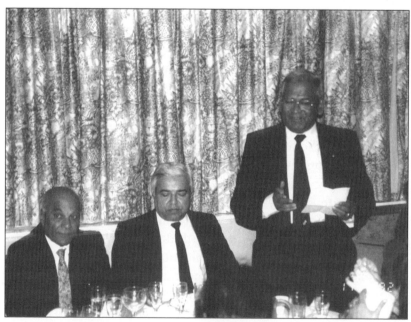

The author (left) with Dr Venogopal (right) and Dr Karim Admani

Stevenson looked across the table at me and asked, 'Dr Chatterjee, I know who you are but who **are** you?' The inference, as I saw it, was that I was not sufficiently important to be negotiating on behalf of the overseas doctors. I was a bit taken aback by such a blunt observation. I looked back at him and answered, 'I'm Dr Chatterjee, a consultant physician, but more importantly I'm the chairman of the Overseas Doctors' Association, elected by around 20,000 practising doctors. But you, sir, were appointed by the BMA.'

While I'm sure my remark didn't go down well with the BMA leader, it certainly elicited a chuckle from one of his colleagues, who blurted out, 'How right you are.' It was Dr Anthony Grabham, BMA's chairman. He was one of the earliest friends I made in the BMA. He was sincere, kind and showed great understanding of the problems of the overseas doctors. A consultant surgeon in Northampton, he was very human and later on became Sir Anthony Grabham. He invited me to give a talk to the BMA and treated me to lunch. I soon discovered that not all in the medical hierarchy were anti-ODA. In fact, quite a few of them were in their own way, some covertly while others quite openly, sympathetic to what we were striving to achieve.

With the right conditions and plenty of support behind it, ODA decided that it would have regular meetings in every large town and city where there were substantial numbers of overseas doctors working. It was also agreed that at every meeting there would be a lecture on an important medical topic to improve or to update the clinical knowledge of those attending. The ODA was now making its presence felt. Both the BMA and the medical hierarchy were taking notice of us. We were firmly on the map.

CHAPTER 14

The medico-political world

EARLY IN 1976 I received the news that the partner of my friend Dr Sunil Bhattacharya had died. Mohini, a divorcée, was living with him when she committed suicide. Her death was a terrible shock to us all, particularly my two daughters, who were very close to her. Mohini, also a doctor, was a delightful person and a joy to be with. The news of her tragic death came at a time when Dr Bhattacharya's involvement with the Overseas Doctors' Association was increasing. The association had decided that he should be in charge of the publication of ODA's *News Review*. The magazine got off to a modest start, as in the early stages of its launch it had no advertisement income of any kind to speak of. It hit trouble when Dr Bhattacharya, in a burst of enthusiasm, wrote an editorial piece that was critical of the Royal College of Physicians in London.

It was my premier college and its registrar took umbrage over the critical comments contained in the piece. He placed the responsibility for its publication squarely at my door and reportedly told the president of the college, Sir Douglas Black, that I had failed to uphold the institution in the high estimation expected of its members and fellows. This simply was not true. I had nothing against my old college. On the contrary, I was as proud of being one of its fellows at that time as I am now. I was unhappy about the unpleasantness the editorial piece had created and wanted to make my position in the matter clear to Sir Douglas, so I sought an urgent meeting with him in London. I made it plain to him that, although I was the chairman of the Overseas Doctors' Association, I was not responsible for the comments contained in the offending article. As a matter of fact I did not agree with the tone and substance of the piece but, that said, I could not interfere with the opinion held and expressed by other members of the association whom I considered perfectly responsible people who understood what they were doing.

However, I regretted that the criticism had caused hurt feeling on both sides. Sir Douglas listened to me patiently and attentively and agreed on almost every point I raised. He said he would have a word with the registrar and promised I would hear no more on the subject from the college. I was pleased I had managed to clear the air but felt aggrieved that the registrar should have chosen not to contact me before taking the matter further and implicating me in it. I seriously wondered if things would have gone as far as they did had I been a local doctor and not one from overseas. As promised by Sir Douglas, I did not hear from the college on the subject again.

ODA was now well-rooted and blooming. Dr Alex Merison, professor of engineering at Bristol University – later Sir Alex Merison when he became its vice-chancellor – invited us to a meeting with him. He was heading an investigation into the National Health Service at the behest of the Government and, as such, his remit included grievances of junior doctors, many of whom were also members of our association. He wanted to include our evidence into the findings of his inquiry. Dr Akram Sayeed, a leading ODA light, produced a document that spelled out our views on the subject. Armed with the document, we went to meet Dr Merison and submitted it for consideration. Our case was simple and straightforward. We wanted to highlight the problems faced by the overseas doctors who formed a sizeable chunk of the NHS medical staff. The feeling was that these doctors had been let down both by the employers and by their own union, the British Medical Association. When the Merison report was published it recommended a whole range of measures which duly addressed the issues we had raised in our document.

Late one night the telephone rang at home. It was Lord Hunt from the House of Lords. He asked me if I knew that the Government was planning a quick remedy for the NHS ills by passing an Enabling Act in the House of Commons. The aim of the Act, from what I could glean from the telephone conversation, was to avoid detailed discussion on the Health Service. My immediate reaction was that it was an unwelcome development and that ODA should oppose it every inch of the way. The matter was later discussed by the ODA executive committee and we agreed to seek the opinion of other active members. But in a later development the Government decided that it would introduce a Bill to alter the Medical Act, but any changes would be incorporated after consultations with the various bodies concerned, including ODA.

ODA membership was rising at a rapid pace. As its work increased it became imperative to appoint a full-time secretary. The association had a competent executive committee but as its members had demanding, full-time jobs the time they had at their disposal for its work was limited, so they met mainly on Saturdays or Sundays, sometimes both. It was increasingly being felt at these meetings that, if ODA wanted to play a more active role, it would need the support of the General Medical Council. But here we were faced with a limitation: none of the GMC members was from overseas. It was therefore imperative that ODA should have some representation on this august body. However, that was possible only if there were elections to the council and candidates from ODA taking part in it were successful at securing seats on it. Along with a few other members, I was convinced that, in order to be effective, we had also to bring about changes from within the system. We had to field candidates for the GMC election whenever it came. At almost every ODA meeting I rammed this point home in the most emphatic terms.

A new Medical Act was being talked about and this offered us a window of opportunity to have discussions with top Government and Opposition health officials, including the Tory spokesman on health, Patrick Jenkin. At these meetings we freely expressed our views. The upshot of all this was that I received a letter from the Health Secretary, Barbara Castle, asking me to meet her in her office. Accompanied by two other members of the ODA executive committee, I went to see her. Mrs Castle had a reputation for being a tough politician to deal with, but we found her most charming and helpful. She listened very carefully to everything we had to say but at the end of it all she made no promises. This, we were later told, was normal practice, as Ministers receiving delegations rarely made any firm commitments on the basis of just one meeting and having heard what in their view was only one side of the argument. A person who greatly helped us at the time was Dr Gerard Vaughan, who later went on to become a Health Minister under the Conservatives.

As these things were moving forward, my domestic situation was also improving. Pet, our second daughter, had qualified as a doctor and her graduation was to be held in Manchester. My wife and I decided to attend the ceremony. How proud I felt when she went up the steps to receive her medical degree. The sight of all those gowned graduates hurrying and scurrying in all directions with cheerfully smiling faces instantly took me back me to the day I received my own degree in Patna all those years ago. The difference was that, despite becoming the first doctor in our family, I had gone all alone to the graduation hall, with no one from the family present to share in my joy or to cheer me. It brought a lump to my throat but it quickly dissolved when my attention was deflected from the past by the joyful activities around us. There was our Pet, looking like an oversized penguin in her black gown, proudly holding her rolled-up certificate in a cardboard tube and waving to us enthusiastically. There were two doctors in the house now and it made me feel ten feet tall.

My research and development programme was going full steam ahead and our demand was growing. I was quite lucky that I could get adequate help and full support from my hospital. I had been given two assistants to help me, one of whom was an Indian doctor. He had written me a letter to inform me that he was from the same medical college as me. He was looking for a break and thought I might be of help to him as all his past efforts had come to nothing. He wasn't the first such case I had come across but I decided to give him a leg up. As I had the sole responsibility for the two assistants, I appointed him to one of the positions. My gesture to help him, I felt, did not go down well with the hospital authorities.

Some time later I regretted giving him the job because, after gaining valuable experience with us, he started looking for a job elsewhere and seemed to be biding his time for the right opportunity to come along. This attitude was clearly reflected in the quality of his work which I found was slipping. So one afternoon I summoned him into my office and told him that I no longer needed his services and he would have to go. My decision to get rid of him clearly annoyed him and he complained to the hospital secretary about it. But I was adamant. I had made a decision and I was sticking to it. I had never taken such a drastic step against any member of my staff before and it left a very bad taste in my mouth for a long time to come.

At ODA I was getting invitations from all over the country to come and speak to members and explain the progress the association was making. We were also invited to visit India. The invitations from the subcontinent, I thought, would provide an excellent opportunity for senior doctors from Britain, both Indian and British, to go to India on lecture tours. ODA was keen to widen its horizons and put in the in-tray the educational needs of its members. I saw it as an important step forward because it made us more than just a pressure group. In reality, we were a group of doctors who had come to Britain to learn and practise medicine. While we did not seek any special favours, we were also against any hurdles being placed in the path to better conditions and chances of promotion. I was happy with the change of direction that ODA was making and was greatly assisted by other senior officials who were now, it was heartening to know, instantly recognisable among the overseas medical fraternity in Britain. But this 'fame' was not without a price tag. The telephone sometimes rang at the most awkward hours at home with the pettiest of complaints and unreasonable requests for favours. Occasionally we were treated as if we were full-time, paid union officials whose only job was to deal with the members' complaints as and when they decided to make them.

It was well known then, as it is known now, that the overseas doctors who went into general practice did so because they were denied opportunities to work in hospitals. Those who did manage to get hospital posts found their promotion route blocked. Medical graduates who qualified from British universities needed to send out three or four applications to secure an interview while for those from overseas the number was four to five times higher. The irony of it was that almost all of them had come to Britain after paying for their graduation and postgraduation levels out of their own pocket – well, at the cost of their parents, really – and Britain was getting them for free, having spent not a single copper

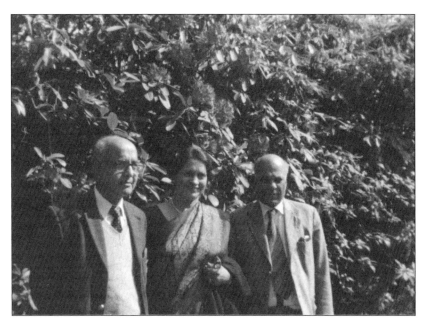

The author (right) in his garden with (left) Dr K. P. Bhargava and Dr Shanta Bhargava in 1981

coin on their education or their training, while the tax payers in Britain picked up the tab for locally-trained doctors, which ran into thousands of pounds and in some cases even more. I felt it was all grossly unfair.

At this period of time in my life there were two dominant things: my hospital work and ODA. Virtually all my time and energies were taken up by them. So, as one can imagine, there were plenty of swings of satisfaction and roundabouts of frustration. In 1977, I received an invitation from Sir John Richardson, president of the General Medical Council, to meet him. He wanted to discuss the problems facing members of our association. I went to see him and explained to him that ODA was not a militant organisation and its members were not card-carrying revolutionaries. They just wanted some improvements in their working conditions and an equal chance on the ladder of promotion. He was extremely sympathetic and promised that he would take our views on board in all future negotiations with the powers that be.

As things proceeded at their own lively pace, the time for GMC elections arrived, the first GMC elections under the

Medical Act 1976. This was the moment that ODA had been waiting for. We wanted our voice to be heard loud and clear within the GMC and the election offered that chance. We fielded seven candidates in the election and worked hard to ensure our success. We sent out hundreds of letters and went round hospitals explaining our policies and canvassing for support. There were no means of knowing how well our campaign had gone but, come the result day, we were pleasantly surprised that four of us, including Dr Admani and myself, were elected to the GMC. It was gratifying to discover later that the two of us were among those who had polled the highest number of votes.

After the formation of the new GMC, I started to attend its meetings every month. This was a demanding task but I was determined that, since it was something that I had chosen to do of my own free volition, I would see it through no matter what. During these meetings we brought it to the council's notice that there were hardly any overseas doctors on the various committees of regional, area and district health authorities. To my great surprise and joy I soon found myself appointed as a member of the North-West Regional Health Authority.

Regional and area health authorities were powerful bodies who were responsible for the medical services within their area. It was here that the region's medical needs and politics met. For me it was the first time I had come into contact with the medico-political world. It is difficult to say whether it was the campaigning work of ODA that led to an increase in the number of its members finding themselves on committees and sub-committees of regional, area and district health authorities or whether these changes were the result of the changing landscape of the British medical world. I suspect it was a combination of both. That the overseas doctors were at last beginning to influence the decision-making processes was a welcome change. I felt happy – certainly satisfied – with the progress we had made so far.

Overseas doctors who came to Britain were, by and large, now settled in their jobs. Some were doing better than others, but then some always do. However, a new phenomenon was now coming to the fore. The overseas doctors, not forgetting other profes-sionals from the new Commonwealth who had made this country their home, were sending their children to the best universities and the top medical schools. So, while the source of doctors from the Indian subcontinent and elsewhere was drying up, a new breed was emerging: British doctors of ethnic origin. Their case was different. They, too, were victims of racial prejudice, but this bias was of a diluted kind, and it was restricted mainly to admission to medical schools and procurement of first jobs. However, fortunately, it was nothing compared to what their parents had experienced. And since they belonged to the generation born and brought up in this country, they considered themselves as British and were ready to fight their corner. ODA briefly took up their cause and found there were people in high places and spheres of influence who were willing to listen to us in this matter. Some of them, in fact, were very sympathetic. Among them was Professor Tomlinson, Professor of Medicine and Dean of Manchester Medical School. He promised that he would do everything in his power to remedy the situation regionally, if not nationally.

In just a few years ODA had achieved most, though by no means all, of its objectives. It had brought various benefits to thousands of overseas doctors working in Britain. It had acted as a guide for them, highlighted their grievances, improved their working conditions, cleared their path to promotion and, most importantly in my opinion, helped bring about a change in the attitude of medical authorities towards them. It could, with reason, give itself a small pat on the back. For me it was time to take my foot off the pedal.

CHAPTER 15

Towards retirement

M Y WORK AT THE HOSPITAL was increasing. I was now in the last quarter of my career as a consultant and it was a frightfully busy time for me – ward rounds, outpatient clinics, research and what have you. My laboratory, which had become a regional institution, was one of the focal points of research into chest diseases and I was quite proud of that fact. I had applied for and obtained a grant from the Regional Health Authority to investigate in detail the management of bronchial asthma using new drugs that were coming on the market. Part of this research was to establish a pattern of treatment for the disease and also to train and involve junior doctors in it.

One of the junior doctors to take part in the project was Akinje Oboneo. A tall, smart, Afro-Caribbean with the looks of a movie star, he had qualified from Manchester University and had applied for a job with us. He was one of the candidates short-listed for an interview. As the interview progressed, I asked him what he wanted to do after he had completed his training with us. He looked straight at me, smiling, as if it was a very simple question to which he knew the answer backwards, and replied in a crisp, confident voice, 'I want to be a professor of medicine and this research project will give an excellent start.' I almost stood up in my seat. Talk of being ambitious! It was a straight answer to a straight question from a very straight man. It also brought a smile to the lips of Dr Leslie Doyle, who was another member of the interviewing panel and was sitting next to me.

Dr Oboneo joined us in due course and worked very diligently for a number of years. When he left, the young doctor had excellent references under his belt. Time wore on until years later I received a letter from Bulawayo, Zimbabwe. It was from Dr Oboneo. He wanted to let me know that he had been appointed senior lecturer in the department of medicine of the university there and was firmly on course to become what he had told us at the interview he wanted to be. When I read the letter, I felt very pleased for him. He deserved to do well in life. Dr Oboneo was one of the brightest sparks I had the chance to work with in my medical career.

One morning, in the course of my daily work routine, I saw a woman of around sixty who had come to see me about her medical problem. She was an old patient of mine and I vaguely remembered having seen her once or twice before. On her last visit she had had an X-ray of her chest taken and, glancing at it, I spotted a sinister-looking shadow, which injected some urgency into her case. I had a brief chat with her and told her that she would have to be admitted straight away. More tests were needed and these would be carried out the following day. I told her that I had already spoken to the thoracic surgeon about the case and that he would also be involved in further investigation. She studied my face for a moment or two and then said, with a note of disappointment in her voice, that she wouldn't be able to comply with my instructions. I felt a trifle vexed by what I read as a point-blank refusal. But I was also curious as to why, despite knowing the seriousness of her case, she was turning down the course of action I had suggested.

'You see, doctor, I've an important appointment later today,' she explained politely. Before I could suggest any alternatives, she asked quite out of the blue, 'Doctor, do you think I'm going to die?'

I could not recall having been asked such a straight question by a patient before. Although I wanted to give a straight answer, I decided to exercise the consultant's prerogative and made my answer evasive. 'My dear, we all have to die some day,' I told her. 'But let's not worry about that. I want to see you in the ward today.'

She reflected on my answer for a time and then said, 'All right, doctor. Not today, but since you've already made arrangements for tests tomorrow, I promise you I'll be here first thing in the morning.'

'Good,' I sighed with relief. 'That'll be just fine.'

'But could you do me a favour?' she asked.

'Go on. What sort of favour?' I inquired.

'I want you to sign a document for me.'

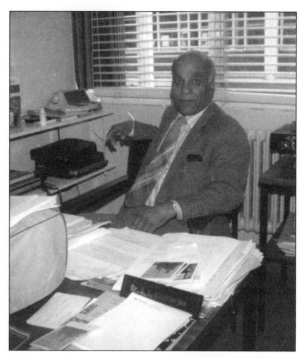

The author in his room at Wythenshawe Hospital

I wasn't quite sure whether I should sign any document that a patient chose to bring, but I told her to bring it anyway and promised I would certainly have a look at it. She went away, renewing her pledge to come back early the next morning. When I turned up for work the following morning, true to her word, she was in the waiting area, talking to a young lad she had brought with her and who was sitting next to her. I had a quick word with her and she introduced me to the boy. After the usual paper work, she was admitted and, accompanied by a nurse, I went to see her in the ward. We exchanged the usual pleasantries and then, with tears swimming in her eyes, she once again asked me if I thought she was going to die.

'Relax,' I told her. 'No need to worry. My colleague will have a look at you later today and we'll discuss your case with him after that.'

Then she reached into her handbag and plucked out a piece of paper and asked me if I'd countersign it after she had put her name to it. I had never witnessed a patient's will before but, as I was only being a witness to her signature, I thought nothing of it. Then she ground down her voice to a whisper and asked me if she could have a word with me strictly in confidence. So I found some small errand for the nurse in order to send her away.

'You know why I wanted to see you, doctor?' she asked.

'No, not really.'

'You know the young boy I introduced to you earlier as my son?'

'Oh, him. Yes, I do.'

'I told you he's my son. But, in fact, he isn't my son.' She stopped for a bit and then added, as if it was an afterthought, 'He's my grandson.'

I didn't read too much into it. Son or grandson, maybe it was just a slip of the tongue or something of that nature and she was just trying to put the facts right.

'My husband had an incestuous relationship with my daughter,' she went on in a solemn tone. 'I found that out when she became pregnant. I reported him to the police and he was sent down for seven and a half years. When my daughter had the baby, I adopted it and sent my girl to London. She's a happily married woman now. Nobody knows about it. Not a soul. I'm leaving all my property and other things to the boy.'

I recalled that in the will, apart from the house, there were other assets of considerable value. It was clear she wanted to make sure that, should something happen to her while she was in hospital, there was enough for the young lad to live on until he was old enough to take care of himself. I found her concern, her sincerity and her honesty truly moving. I patted her on the shoulder to show my admiration for what she was doing, while my mind took my imaginary cap off to her. What anguish! What suffering! What sacrifice!

That night I had a telephone call from the ward sister, informing me that the patient had died in bed. What deliverance.

My research project on asthma was now almost complete and I thought it was time to start thinking in terms of having a postgraduate conference on the results. I sounded out the plan on my colleagues and their response was very positive and encouraging. Not only were they in favour of a conference, some even offered to help me in organising it. Dr Leslie Doyle, one of the senior consultants in the hospital, threw his full weight behind the proposal. The two of us along with a handful of others had a series of meetings to thrash out a programme and submitted it to the regional authority. I contacted the professor of medicine at Manchester University and the president of the Royal College of Physicians in London, Sir Douglas Black, who in the past had always been helpful and encouraging. I also got in touch with the chief medical officer of the region and he agreed to chair one of the sessions.

The day of the conference arrived – the culmination of weeks and months of planning and preparation. I had in the past attended scores of conferences and thought nothing of it. In medicine they are part of your continuing education. But for my own I was full of trepidation, wondering how things would turn out in the end. Delegates from all over the country as well as from the Continent were present, eminent specialists in their fields. The morning session passed off without a hitch or glitch, so smoothly, in fact, that secretly I felt proud of my organisational skills. After lectures and talks from well-known doctors in the morning session, we had lunch with glasses of wine and settled down for the afternoon session. It got under way as it was planned to do. Sir Douglas was in the chair and Dr Oboneo was speaking on the findings of our research when we heard a loud, thudding noise in the hall. It was followed by what sounded like interrupted snoring. Lights, which had been dimmed for the lecture, were put full on and we found Dr Aron Holtzel, a speaker who had earlier given an excellent lecture, collapsed on the floor. A number of doctors rushed to help him, only to discover that he had suffered a massive heart attack. We tried to resuscitate him but he died. Dr Holtzel was a specialist in paediatric chest diseases in Manchester and had spent his life practising medicine in the United Kingdom and Europe. The conference broke up in disarray and sad confusion. We didn't know what to do. There was plenty of sympathy for the family of the deceased and to a lesser degree for me whose conference had suddenly come to an end in such a sorry way. None of the delegates had had an experience like this in their lives and never wanted it to happen in the future. As I was the chief organiser of the event, the heart-breaking task of going to Dr Holtzel's house in Sale, Cheshire, to break the news to the family fell to me.

Time slipped by and soon I found that I was fast approaching my retirement. I told the hospital that I would be hanging up my stethoscope in the middle of 1987. I also made it known to the hospital and my department that I wanted no farewell. Farewells, to my mind, are never happy occasions, especially for those whose farewell it is. Goodbyes, in any case, are not in my nature. I see them as signifying the end of something. I think life is a great continuum. When one thing ends, another surfaces or something that's already there takes its place. It's all a bit like a jack-in-the-box. You thump one thing down and while your eyes are still on it another leaps up. Maybe it's these beliefs, these subtle nuances of personality that make us what we are. Nothing good, bad or indifferent about them. No moral dilemmas. Just individual preferences and small differences with others. I knew some of my colleagues would be sorry to see me go. Then on the other hand maybe some would be glad to see the back of me. In my experience that is so in a vast number of cases. I also forewarned my colleagues that, if a surprise party was sprung on me, I'd decline to take part in it. But in spite of all that I was invited to some private dinners. These were, of course, more of an informal nature – people sitting around the table scoffing wine, tucking into meat and vegetables, sipping coffee and munching mints and leisurely chatting about life's little and big things, though coming towards the end of one's working life did invariably creep into it.

On the last working day I had just finished the morning session when Paulette Davis, who had joined the clinic as a bright-eyed, fresh-faced young nurse and had, by hard work, dedication and a pleasant temperament, risen to become sister in charge, told me not to go on the lunch break my usual way as some repair and refurbishment work had started in one of the corridors and part of the section had been closed off. Instead she recommended that I go through the main out-patients' waiting area. Such a helpful suggestion. I naturally heeded her advice. As I entered the hall I was blown away by the sight of all my staff, colleagues, doctors who had once worked with me and, of course, a handful of patients lying in wait for me. Obviously, my colleagues had thrown all my warnings out of the window and gone ahead with the farewell. Confronted by a large gathering, I was not angry; merely amused. All sorts of emotions were working inside me – gratitude for my staff, sincerity towards my patients, humility for myself. There was Dr Doyle, who had already retired, along with several former colleagues. And so began the farewell I did not want. Bravely I stood there, at times embarrassed by the glowing words said about me. Quietly whirring was a video camera which moved from face to face and person to person, recording the proceedings and the reactions of those present. From time to time I cast an eye around and spotted a misty-eyed secretary here and a sniffling nurse there, the people I had dealings with on a daily basis. I was deeply touched.

Speakers sang the praises of my services to the hospital in glowing terms and I felt grateful to those who were lavishing the tributes, underscoring the work that I had done and recalling some funny work-related incident, the odd anecdote in which I figured as a hero. Standing there before the gathering, my mind raced back to the first morning I had gone to work at Baguley Hospital. Clearly feeling a bit nervous, I had failed to take notice of the 'No Entry' sign and was driving along when I was waved down by a doctor in a white coat who pointed out my folly to me and followed it up by a mild rebuke. Now, more than thirty years later, I would shortly be leaving Wythenshawe Hospital – even the hospital had undergone a name change – for the last time and driving the right way. I thought I would probably come back as a visitor, a patient, even a well-wisher to someone else's farewell, but not as a consultant. After the farewell speeches and toasts and presentations I went back to my lab, mumbling and grumbling to myself in an undertone, and sparked a mini farewell there. All manner of good wishes were expressed and a whole series of pats on the back and handshakes followed. When the whole *tamasha* was over, I gathered my paraphernalia in bags I had collected over the years at medical conferences, headed to my car and drove straight home.

Hung over from the goodbyes, I made myself a cup of tea and sat down in my favourite chair, gently rocking back and forth, going over the varied panorama of my busy, humdrum life – from a young lad playing cricket with makeshift bats and wickets in the mangroves of Patna, India, to a consultant physician in England and a former chairman of this, that and the other organisation, battling to improve the lot of overseas doctors, promoting race relations in the city in which I lived, passing judgment in court on a bewildering variety of cases. One case that was forever fresh in my mind concerned a young man who was charged with indecent exposure – at a blind people's home. I wanted to let him go with a warning because I felt exposing his private parts in the bone-chilling draught of a frosty morning was in itself punishment enough, but I had to slap a fine on him in keeping with the offence. In another case, a father refused to pay maintenance money to his children because a large chunk of his income went on having his toupees dry-cleaned during an exceptionally hot summer. Sipping the lukewarm tea, I also thought of my family. Petula had acquired a busy general practice in Wythenshawe while at the same time she worked as a clinical assistant in

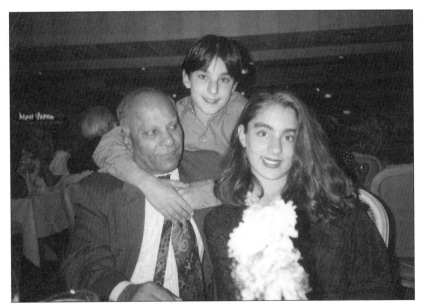

The author with Ruth and Tom in 1992

hospital. Camille was a community nurse in Nottingham and the mother of two teenage children. My wife had been a senior medical social worker for a number of years. Between us, we had well served the medical needs of the community of which we were a part.

When the mellow mood and introspection were over and the unfinished Darjeeling tea had gone cold, reality tiptoed back. But it hadn't returned to ruin my private party. Just the opposite. I thought to myself that I was only sixty-five and fit and well, with plenty of get-up-and-go. My working life may have drawn to a close but I could still do a lot. Leaving the stage didn't mean the wings were out of reach. So it was time for a shift in gear and a slight swerve in direction. I was ready to reinvent myself, seek a new incarnation.

CHAPTER 16

A debt of gratitude

THE FIRST FEW DAYS of retirement were a period of blissful relaxation and mellow fruitfulness. Early rising, toast on the hoof and frantic dashes out of the house with the briefcase were a thing of the past, albeit of the most recent past. Now I could afford the supreme luxury of doing one thing at one time and give it the attention it deserved. Cooked breakfast, with steam rising from the plate, and at a table, was a totally new experience and a thoroughly enjoyable one at that. To have the morning newspaper by the side of the teapot was sheer luxury. What was to come after it merited little thought over what was already on the table. It came soon enough anyway. Although my private practice was still there, I could afford to stand by the French window of the lounge and watch the raindrops dance on the pane before forming tiny rivulets and disappearing into the woodwork. Hitherto I had seen the rain falling mostly on the car windscreen to and from work and it was the wipers that dispersed it. The trees swaying in the wind, birds hopping on the hedge, the leaping green of the grass and the vivid yellow of the flowers – retirement was truly reaching the parts that had not been touched before. With a feeling of satisfaction, I was also able to survey the family scene at leisure.

Pet, my younger daughter, was married and had a little boy, Nicholas. Camille's two children, Tom and Ruth, were grown up and attending university – Tom was in Sheffield while Ruth grappled with media studies at Liverpool. She had also acquired a boyfriend. Nicholas was the latest addition and I was quite involved with him because Pet lived close to us and I had time on my hands to help her and to play with the young 'un. Our son Nigel had finished his accountancy course and was ready to settle into a career. We were looking forward to it with eager anticipation when one day he sprang a surprise on us by announcing that he was off to Bermuda. His company had

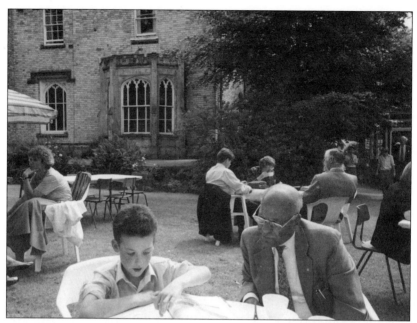

The author with grandson Nicholas aged 8 at his Prep School on Prize-giving Day

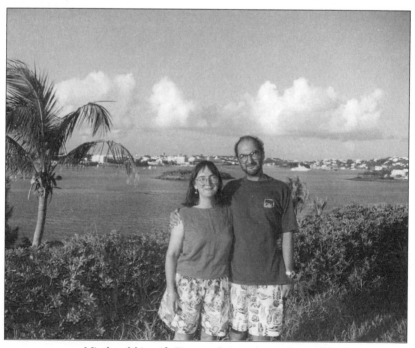

Nigel and his wife Fran in their garden in Bermuda

decided to send him there as an expert on insolvency. We were happy with his rapid progress, and happy to learn that he would soon be a director, but sad at the same time that he would no longer be just a few minutes' drive away from us. I knew I would miss him, as he was my guide and my counsel on many subjects.

But while these leisurely-paced pursuits continued, my inner voice kept telling me to make the most of them as they were not going to last a long time. And, believe me, one's inner voice is seldom wrong. Barely a few weeks into retirement, I received a telephone call from Dr Karim Admani, who was now chairman of the Overseas Doctors' Association. He, along with his deputy, Dr S Venogopal, wanted to come and see me about some business connected with the association and so we fixed a date for the meeting. The two of them arrived on my doorstep on the agreed morning and revealed, over a cup of tea, that they were having problems with the magazine, the ODA *News Review*. As the duo reeled out the litany of problems, they suggested that, as I had free time on my hands, I should help them out by getting involved with the magazine and putting it on an even keel. The association's financial state, I was told, was far from healthy and, that being the case, it could not afford to inject any cash into the publication. In short, their message was clear: take over the magazine, somehow make it work and expect nothing from us. Well, thank you fellows, I do have some fine friends!

Time was another commodity in short supply. We had to act and act fast to get the next edition out while at the same time work out a long-term strategy to make the whole thing viable. As the *News Review*'s future was at stake, any quick-fix, on-the-spot decision on my part was out of the question. I sent the two away with the promise that I'd give the matter my most serious consideration. I needed first to sort things out in my mind. A couple of days later I had a serious, heart-to-heart discussion with Enid over the magazine's future. Surprisingly, she showed plenty of enthusiasm for breathing new life into the ailing publication.

While I was thinking about what I'd do if I decided to get involved with the venture, it was brought to my notice that James Lewis, a stalwart at *The Guardian* who had past connections with India and had also been to the subcontinent to train Indian journalists, was about to leave the newspaper. This was heaven-sent for both the magazine and me. Without a second thought I approached him with the request to take over the editorship of the *News Review*. He very kindly agreed. Round about that time my secretary at the hospital, Ann Wood, was also coming towards her retirement. When I got in touch with her she, too, showed willingness to join us on part-time basis. Mrs Wood, a pleasant and efficient secretary, was the sort of person who can be an instant asset to any organisation the minute they walk into it. More than that, she was willing to learn, because when I told her I didn't like dictating into tape-recording machines she went and joined evening classes to brush up her shorthand.

The team building had started and was proceeding smoothly. Cash was the next big hurdle to cross. Once again I turned to my old, trusted friend, Patrick Knowlson, and to Mike Gatenby. They were heads of two large pharmaceutical companies and agreed to help me but with a warning that it wouldn't be easy producing a serious, responsible medical magazine. Help also came from Mr Glen Williams, director of another large drug firm,

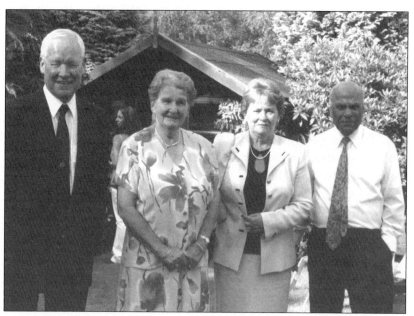

(left to right) Dr Patrick Knowlson, Enid, Mrs Nora Knowlson, the author

who agreed to advertise in the *News Review*. I soon realised to my great delight that I could muster six full pages of advertisements. Then there were other bits and bobs. This was more than enough to cover the costs.

James Lewis found a suitable printer in Manchester, Roberts and Co. Run by two young brothers, John and David Roberts, it was a small, personal firm, ideal for our needs. I now had an editor, a secretary, a printer and sufficient resources to get a few editions out. Next I approached a number of medical feature writers and other specialists and they agreed to contribute on a regular basis. An eager and willing hand in all this was my wife. Enid started attending medical meetings as a jotter for Mr Lewis. She made copious notes, interviewed people and got quotes to put flesh on stories. With help coming from so many quarters, we got every issue of the magazine out on its due date. The money it raised also went some way towards organising the association's annual conference and dinner in London, an important and colourful occasion in Britain's medical calendar. I was pleased being at the heart of all this, playing a significant role.

Amid this fresh burst of activity I felt that the association was once again gradually taking over my life. A lot of my time was

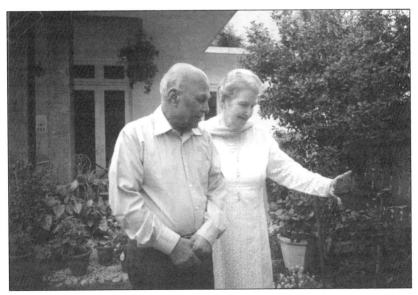

The author and Enid in the garden of Dr Shanta Bhargava's home in New Delhi

taken up procuring advertisements for the magazine and chasing medical writers; there were endless rounds of meetings and travelling up and down the country to collect material. And, on top of that, this time it wasn't just confined to me. Demands on my wife's time were also growing. Telephone calls at home connected with the magazine became more frequent and longer. The association, too, was undergoing a change with the arrival of young blood. There were rumblings over the style and contents of the *News Review*, and disagreements between some members and office bearers, hitherto below the surface, became quite open and their frequency also increased. Like an ill-tempered puppy clinging to the ankles and refusing to let go, these problems had their negative side which, as time went on, wore me down and I began to feel the strain. So I decided it was time to take a back seat or, preferably, no seat at all. My wife shared this view with me. Therefore, when the first opportunity presented itself to us we both bowed out of our roles and pushed off to India for a well-deserved holiday and to attend the wedding of one of my nephews in Calcutta.

An annual trip to India was fast becoming something of a enjoyable habit with me. I was pleased that my wife shared this enthusiasm with equal fervour. For a start there were Drs Kamta and Shanta Bhargava and their family to meet in New Delhi. Then I had my brother and his clan to visit in Patna. There were also new things to see and new places to go to and old things and old places to see in a new light. During one of the trips an interesting thing happened. I chanced to meet Professor A. K. N. Sinha, professor of medicine at Patna Medical College and president of the Indian Medical Council, whom I had recently met. On a visit to Britain in 1988, he was staying at the house of Dr Madan Gupta, a general practitioner in Oldham, Lancashire, when I was visiting Dr Gupta on some business. We were introduced and we talked about our alma mater. During this somewhat brief meeting, the professor told me he was interested in promoting postgraduate work in India with the co-operation of doctors from Britain. He had even approached the government of India with proposals to set up a fund under the auspices of the Indian Medical Council. The fund would pay for the conferences, seminars and other meetings at which the visiting doctors from Britain would speak. I told him it was an excellent idea and had my whole-hearted support. I also informed him that I had taken groups of doctors to various part of Britain for postgraduate conferences and once even to the Egyptian capital of Cairo. That trip had proved to be a memorable one not only because of the significant number of doctors who took part in it and the high quality of the papers they presented on their chosen subjects, but also for the sightseeing that followed once the conference was over and done with. On the social itinerary were visits to Aswan Dam and the pyramids.

So when I met Professor Sinha in New Delhi the following year, the subject of doctors from Britain visiting India came up again. I was accompanied by Dr Venogopal and also present at the meeting in the Indian capital were a number of high-ranking officials from the Ministry of Health. We were told that the Prime Minister of India at the time, Mr P. V. Narasimha Rao, had been told of the project and was keen on it. A meeting with him was hurriedly arranged and I went to see him in his office. Talking with him on the subject was like preaching to the converted. The Prime Minister agreed to initiate discussions between the Health Ministry and the Indian Medical Council to take things forward. Within a matter of weeks we learned from the council that the project had been given the go-ahead and that funds had been made available to the council to invite medical experts from the United Kingdom to lecture in India.

I took this new venture seriously and back in Britain suggested that we form a separate body to handle it. Following detailed discussions on the subject, the Indo-British Medical Co-operation Committee came into being. One of the main tasks of the committee was to pick senior physicians and surgeons to travel to India for a week or ten days and speak at universities and medical colleges on their speciality and on any recent advances that had been made in their field. As the funds at the disposal of the Indian Medical Council were limited, the doctors from the United Kingdom were required to pay their own air fare between Britain and India while the host institutions were expected to pick up the tab for board and lodging, as well as travel within the subcontinent.

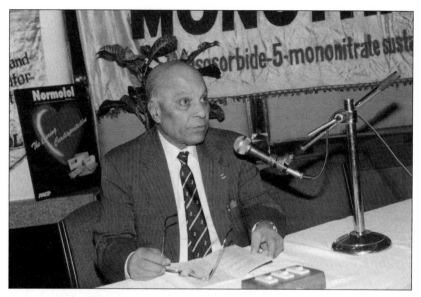

The author lecturing at a medical symposium in 1995

We were lucky to obtain the services of such eminent experts as Dr Colin Bray, consultant cardiologist from Manchester, Dr Penny Chandiok, senior consultant in Genito-Urinary Medicine at Withington Hospital in Manchester, Mr Ali Rehman, consultant cardio-thoracic surgeon at Wythenshawe Hospital, Dr Mohinder Singh Gill, consultant cardiologist from London, Dr Umesh Prabhu, consultant paediatrician, Bury, Dr Mohinder Chopra, consultant physician from Tamesside, Dr Venkat Mani, consultant physician, Wigan, and Dr Jeffrey Wade, consultant cardiologist at Manchester Royal Infirmary.

On each trip we took four consultants to India. Dr Chandiok gladly volunteered to lecture on her subject which also embraced Aids, a disease which has acquired special significance in the Indian context as it poses a major threat to the subcontinent's vast population in the coming years. This is the sort of valuable contribution the Co-operation Committee made to the world of medicine in India. My experience was that whoever we approached to share their knowledge with their Indian counterparts showed a keen interest in the project. It was only their previous commitments that prevented some of them from taking part in the experiment.

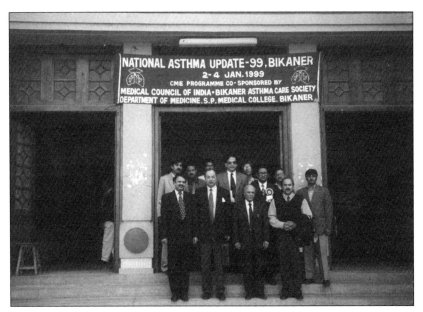

In Bikaner with participants in the 1999 CME programme

Lecturing in far-flung corners of the subcontinent involved a lot of travel – from Patna in the East to Trivandrum and Madras in the South, Bombay and Poona in the West and Delhi and Bikaner in the North. The Bikaner visit where our host was Professor Abdul Mohammed was very interesting. We had three days there and concentrated on medicine, surgery and gynaecology. Bikaner lies at the edge of Rajasthan's desert and we travelled by train, covering a vast chunk of the desert. There were other cities, too, such as Calcutta, Indore and Gauhati. The postgraduate meeting in Trivandrum concentrated on tuberculosis and genito-urinary medicine. Here, Dr Chandiok took charge of the sessions on GU medicine which lasted three days.

I have always believed that the doctors who had come to work and settle in Britain had had their basic medical education in India at great expense to themselves, their family and the country at large. Some had gone on to obtain postgraduate degrees. They had then dispensed the hard-earned knowledge they had acquired in the land in which they had decided to settle. I thought they owed something to the country of their birth and their education and the least they could give as pay-back was the benefit of their experience to those who were coming behind them. I think that after parents, teachers and lecturers who teach you have the most profound influence on your life. To this day I remember many of my teachers who taught me, from the basic three Rs to more complicated subjects like physiology and biochemistry. I was quite willing to pay back my debt of gratitude and, I'm glad to say, so were many – virtually all, really – that we got in touch with. Dr Penny Chandiok thought that sentiments aside, in the ever-shrinking, inter-dependent world of the twenty-first century, the flow of knowledge between nations, especially in the field of science, technology and medicine, should be a multi-lane highway. All in all we made eighteen trips to India and I would like to think the committee contributed a fair bit in the exchange of knowledge in its small way.

The century, and indeed the millennium, were slowly drawing to a close. Although there was still plenty of time left, people were turning their thoughts to how they would usher in the third millennium. Some were talking of outlandish schemes of going to New Zealand to be among the first in the world to see the dawn of the twenty-first century. Others were more modest in their approach and just wanted to be in some big city like London or Paris with friends to mark the occasion. My plans, among other things, included bringing my commitments to the ODA to an end. I had been associated with it for over a quarter of a century. So at the association's annual conference at Manchester in 1999, I announced that I was retiring. Many expressed surprise, some wanted me to stay on and others praised the work I had done for the overseas doctors over the years. Resolute in my decision, I waved to the applauding delegates and brought my ODA and ODA *News Review* chapters finally to a close.

CHAPTER 17

The last syllable

RETIRING FROM MEDICAL PRACTICE did not mean that I lost
touch with everything with which I was previously involved. The Indian Association, which figured so highly in my
life in the past, continues to do so, now that I have more time on
my hands. Every Sunday I go there for a couple of hours –
sometimes longer – when the Hindu Society holds a prayer
meeting there. It is usually well attended with many familiar faces
around. After *puja*, a simple, vegetarian meal is served, as food is
considered to be an important part of praying. When that is over,
people mix and mingle freely with each other. I am not a person
with strong, deep-rooted religious beliefs and as such it is
socialising that appeals to my fancy and takes me there. Problems
of a general nature, like law and order, the Health Service,
military conflicts, the rising cost of living, political shenanigans of
the major parties, are usually discussed by those who attend,
though superficially and not at any great length. But at times the
problems are more specific and of a personal nature. Some seek
advice and I put forward my suggestions. People are quite civil
and polite about it. They listen attentively but whether they
follow them or not is an altogether different matter.

I have also become involved with two new organisations – the
Bengali Cultural Group and the Ramakrishna Mission. The main
activity of the first is to organise *Durga Puja*, which is a five-day
annual event, celebrated mainly by the people of Bengal and those
from the eastern region of India, although everyone takes part in
one or the other activity. The festival is held mainly in the
autumn and comprises prayer meetings, social and cultural events
and, yes, food. In October 2004, sadly, the celebrations had to be
abruptly cut short due to a fire which broke out at the Gandhi
Hall and partly destroyed it. I was woken up early in the morning
by a telephone call from the caretaker of the hall who told me
about the blaze and the damage it had caused. I dashed out and

got to the hall as quickly as I could. It broke my heart to see the badly damaged building which had, just a few weeks earlier, undergone extensive renovation and refurbishment costing thousands of pounds, including a brand new floor, a stage of near-professional standard and all the rest.

While the Bengali Cultural Group is a relatively recent entity, Ramakrishna Mission proudly boasts an existence spanning more than 100 years and across 139 centres worldwide. When started in 1897 the Ramakrishna movement had a dozen or so Hindu monks and practically no assets of any kind. But not only did it survive, it seemingly prospered. It is a movement that doesn't convert people from one religion to another but asks them to go to the root of their own religion, whatever it preaches, and take that route to reach God and not by merely talking about Him. It is a movement for peace, tolerance and brotherhood. It preaches selfless service. In India the mission is very active in the field of education, building schools, colleges, hospitals and orphanages. Its most famous son was Swami Vivekanand. Unfortunately, the scope of the mission's branch in the United Kingdom, which is based at Bolton, is somewhat limited, as the medical and educational problems in India are quite different from those in this country.

Retirement has also encouraged me to travel much more frequently and my wife and I go to India at every opportunity that comes our way. Sometimes we create an opportunity ourselves and the duration of our visits has grown longer. In Calcutta, we stay with the Ruia family. Govind Ruia, originally from that neck of the wood but later a successful textile magnate in Manchester, was a good friend of mine and a founding father of the Indian Association. My association with the family goes back a long way. Although Mr Ruia died nearly twenty years ago, my love and affection for the family remain as strong as ever.

There is also my brother Sona, one year my senior, and his daughter Stella in Patna. It is always a delight to visit them and renew old bonds. My brother has followed with keen interest my progress from a skinny little school kid to a hospital consultant in the United Kingdom and the rest. Being on old stamping ground brings back a lot of memories, a whole treasure chest of them, now, of course, pleasantly tinged with nostalgia. I am pleased that

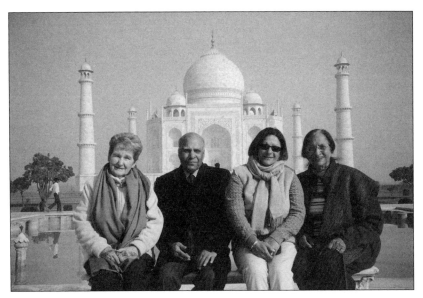

The author with Enid, Petula, and Shanta Bhargava at the Taj Mahal in February 2005

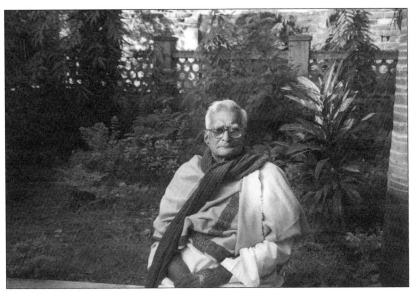

The author's brother, Sona Chatterjee

my wife is also there to share these 'down-memory-lane' trips with me and we often recall, with much amusement, a trip we made to Patna in 1980 when my alma mater was celebrating its golden jubilee – fifty years of service to British India and then the independent state. I had been invited to be the honorary guest on the occasion and it was indeed a proud thing for me to be asked to attend in that capacity. I had been allotted two main tasks: to perform the college's flag-raising ceremony first and then to speak at the postgraduate seminar.

My wife and I packed our bags and flew from London to New Delhi where we changed planes and took the flight to Patna. When the plane touched down in Lucknow, its first stop en route, we were told that the airport at Patna had been shut down because an earlier aircraft had burst one of its tyres on landing. It meant that our plane would be diverted to Ranchi, some 200 miles away. We would disembark there and wait for further instructions. Obviously, we had little say in the matter. The plane took us to Ranchi where we disembarked in the evening. It was a small airport, scarcely bigger than a cricket field with a pavilion. It had strictly limited facilities and my guess was there were no provisions of any kind for night take-offs.

It was clear to me that we were in deep, deep trouble. Alarm bells were ringing and getting louder with each passing minute. My flag-raising ceremony, my lecture at the seminar, my role as the honorary guest all began to fade away from the mind's horizon. The whole trip from Manchester to Patna seemed a complete waste of time, money and effort. Also in some trouble was a group of French tourists who were visiting places of religious and historical interests in Bihar. They had, I learned from one of them, a fairly busy and therefore tight schedule, which included sites such as the ancient tree under which Buddha achieved his nirvana. As I stood there wondering what to do, hands hanging helplessly at my side, I spotted a small, private plane land and taxi to one side. The pilot clambered out of the cockpit and went into the terminal for a few minutes. He talked cursorily to one or two officials and was soon back at the controls and on the runway for the off. My spirits rose. In a wild fit of optimism I thought 'maybe the airline will lay on a special aircraft just like this plane to fly us all to Patna.' Some hope! The evening slowly turned into night and whatever little activity there was at the airport came to a complete halt.

The French visitors, or their tour guide, eager to get on with the sightseeing business, had in the meantime managed to hire a coach and, knowing our predicament, very kindly asked if we would like a ride with them to Patna as there was plenty of spare room on the coach. I leapt at the chance although I still had a feeling that we would not be able to make it in time for the morning flag-raising ceremony and my lecture that was to follow shortly afterwards. Everyone, without exception, was starving and the coach driver assured us that around midnight he would stop at a 'lovely' restaurant on the way. My doubts about the salubrious nature of the restaurant were soon confirmed when the coach came to a halt outside a ramshackle roadside eating place, popularly known in India as a *dhaba*, with just some simple curry and chapattis on the menu. But at least it had some food to offer. We thankfully accepted whatever there was and were soon on our way to Patna.

Wonder of wonders, the coach made the college in time. I had a quick shower and a change and was ready to face what I knew would be a long, busy and, in one sense, remarkable day for me. When the VIPs started arriving a few minutes later we were told that the small plane we had seen at Ranchi airport had been sent by the State Governor especially to pick us up, but the pilot somehow missed us and, blissfully unaware that he had come for us, we missed the pilot. As they say, all's well that ends well. My lecture was received with some approval and I was very proud to raise the college flag on the occasion of its golden jubilee. All day, every eye was on me wherever I went, whatever I did, and I enjoyed every minute of it.

Early in July 2002, Ruth, my granddaughter, friend, philosopher, critic, and companion for walks in the park, returned from a holiday in Florida with her boyfriend Dean whom she had met while doing media studies at Liverpool University. Radiant with delight, she took her grandmother quietly into the kitchen and told her that she had something to show her. Moments later I joined them. Ruth, very happy and all aglow, just wouldn't stop smiling, like someone who has a pleasant secret and is dying to share it. From her pocket she pulled out a little box with a blue, velvet cover, opened it and revealed a glinting diamond ring.

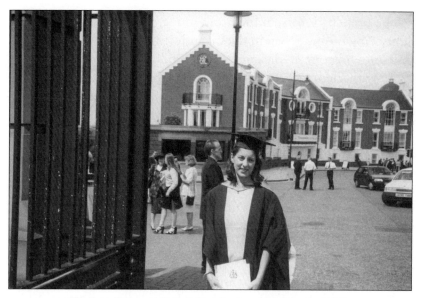

Ruth at Liverpool University after her graduation in 2000

'This is what Dean gave me when he asked me to marry him,' she said and looked at us both for reaction. Of course I was delighted and so was my wife, who said, 'Oh, I'm so pleased for you,' and hugged her, eyes moist with tears of joy.

The wedding was to take place in November 2003, a busy time for getting married, or maybe it only seemed so that year. Everyone in the family was buzzing with excitement. Ruth's parents, Camille and Paul, were understandably anxious that the occasion should be trouble-free, with no last-minute hitches and hiccups. To ensure that, top-level family conferences were held at which duties and responsibilities were allocated. To me was assigned the most enjoyable of roles: having a thunderingly good time with no specific task to do or oversee – a sort of Minister without Portfolio.

Ruth and Dean wanted to get married in Yorkshire and after a trawl of the venues for the occasion, Ruddings Park Hotel, near Harrogate, was chosen. It was an ideal location, surrounded by acres of green land, a lake, stream and deer and other animals roaming freely around as if in their natural habitat. So it was at this idyllic location that we all gathered – friends, well-wishers and relatives, including Nigel and his wife Fran from Bermuda.

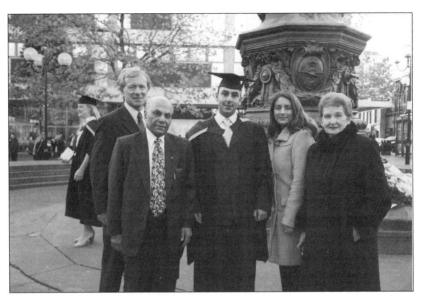

Tom's graduation from Sheffield University in 2001: (from left) Tom's father Paul, the author, Tom, Ruth, Enid

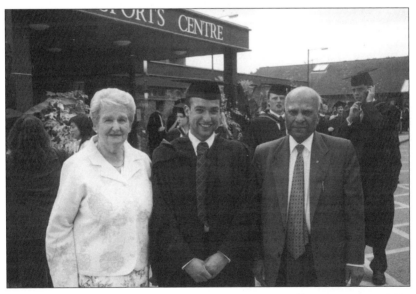

Nicholas and his grandparents after his graduation from Nottingham University in 2004

Guests came from places as far away as Australia, India, America and Europe and, of course, from towns and cities nearer home for a pre-wedding feast. It was a great sight to see so many of them enjoying themselves with everything aplenty, food, drinks, music and dance.

Next day we got up early to prepare ourselves for the big occasion. Everyone spruced up and seemed relaxed, though I suspected that, despite all the thinking and the planning by both sets of parents and other main players, some last-minute nervousness was beginning to creep in. This, I thought, was only natural. After breakfast, we gathered in the hall where the wedding ceremony was to take place. The young couple had decided against a church wedding. At midday, the bride arrived on the arm of her father and walked slowly to the podium where she sat next to the groom. Solemnly, the two took the marriage vows and signed the register. What an exciting time it was – two young people tying the knot in front of more than 200 guests who mattered to them. Brides on their wedding day are always a pleasant sight to behold and I thought Ruth, the little blonde girl who had so often accompanied me on walks, looked stunning on her big day. When the formal part of the wedding was over we

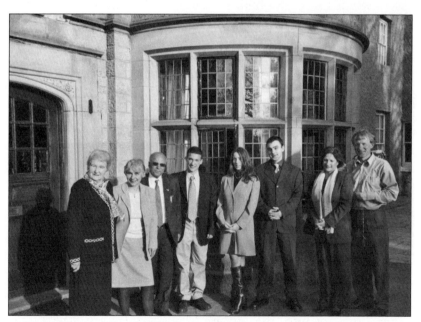

A family group: (from left) Enid, Camille, the author, Nicholas, Ruth, Tom, Petula, Paul

headed for the reception and the merry-making. The reception was one continuous jolly affair and it went on until the early hours when, tired and exhausted, I retired to bed.

Next morning we waved off the newly-married couple as they left for the Maldives on their honeymoon and to start their life together. One by one the guests departed amid foamy farewells and repeated promises to meet again soon. Pet, my younger daughter, travelled with us back to Manchester and kept up an excited chant of how wonderfully happy each part of the wedding had been and the rocking-chair ease with which the whole event had passed off.

A steady drizzle falls outside in the garden. It's a cold morning and a fine film of steam has formed on the glass inside. The telephone rings.

'Grandee, how did it go at Nottingham?'

It's Ruth, wanting to know about the graduation ceremony of my second grandson, Nicholas.

'Fine, just fine. Everything went swimmingly well.'

I tell her all the details. I have seen these ceremonies many times, when my own children graduated and again when Tom and Ruth received their degrees.

Who do I thank for all these happy yesterdays? The woman of twenty-four who bore me as her third child in India or the young girl from Birmingham in her early twenties who said 'yes' when I proposed to her? My grandson, Tom, when he was a nipper crawling on his knees, used to say 'Ces, grandee, ces' because he hadn't yet learned to pronounce 'yes' properly. I think my thanks will go to the 'ces' girl.

Not long ago, I received the shocking news of the death of Dr Karim Admani, a dear friend and a pillar of support to me in the formation of the Overseas Doctors' Association. Our friendship went back more than twenty years during which we had some wonderful times together crusading to improve the lot of foreign medics working in this country. He was a man of spirit, a real fighter. I went to the cemetery in Sheffield where I saw his coffin being lowered into the grave. I wanted to say something, probably to salute him, but, like most of the other mourners, I picked up some soil, slowly poured it over the coffin and wished him a silent goodbye.

A lot of my work is done and with a certain degree of satisfaction. As the sun sets and the evening star appears over my horizon, I'm waiting for 'one clear call' as I set out to sea and praying to my friends and family that there be no 'moaning' in the bar.

Meanwhile, though, it will soon be time for a game of bridge at the club but before I make my way there I must catch my siesta. Could someone please turn the television volume down and slide the stool under my feet?